Complexity Leadership

Nursing's Role in Health-Care Delivery

SECOND EDITION

Diana M. Crowell, PhD, RN, NEA-BC
Nursing Leadership and Education Consultant
Kittery, Maine

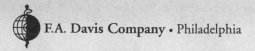
F.A. Davis Company • Philadelphia

F. A. Davis Company
1915 Arch Street
Philadelphia, PA 19103
www.fadavis.com

Printed in the United States of America

Last digit indicates print number: 10 9 8 7 6 5 4 3 2 1

Publisher, Nursing: Joanne Patzek DaCunha, RN, MSN
Acquisitions Editor, Nursing: Susan Rhyner
Director of Content Development: Darlene D. Pedersen, MSN, APRN, BC
Content Project Manager: Christina L. Snyder
Design and Illustration Manager: Carolyn O'Brien

As new scientific information becomes available through basic and clinical research, recommended treatments and drug therapies undergo changes. The author(s) and publisher have done everything possible to make this book accurate, up to date, and in accord with accepted standards at the time of publication. The author(s), editors, and publisher are not responsible for errors or omissions or for consequences from application of the book, and make no warranty, expressed or implied, in regard to the contents of the book. Any practice described in this book should be applied by the reader in accordance with professional standards of care used in regard to the unique circumstances that may apply in each situation. The reader is advised always to check product information (package inserts) for changes and new information regarding dose and contraindications before administering any drug. Caution is especially urged when using new or infrequently ordered drugs.

Library of Congress Cataloging-in-Publication Data

Crowell, Diana M., author.
  Complexity leadership : nursing's role in health care delivery / Diana M. Crowell. -- 2nd edition.
    p. ; cm.
  Includes bibliographical references and index.
  ISBN 978-0-8036-4529-5
  I. Title.
  [DNLM: 1. Nurse Administrators. 2. Leadership. 3. Nurse's Role. 4. Nursing--organization & administration. 5. Nursing, Supervisory. WY 105]
  RT89
  362.17'3068--dc23
                          2015014097

CONTRIBUTORS

Beth Boynton, RN, MS
Nurse Consultant and Author
Portsmouth, New Hampshire

Laura J. Coleman, MPA, MS, RN, CNL
University of New Hampshire
Durham, New Hampshire

Karen Decker-Gendron, MA, MS, CAGS, RN, CNL
Clinical Nurse Leader
Concord Hospital Family Health
  Center
Concord, New Hampshire

Bronwyn Field, RN, MS, CNL
Registered Nurse
Elliot Health System
Manchester, New Hampshire

Emily Fraser Kilroy, BSN, RN
Family Nurse Practitioner Student
University of New Hampshire
Durham, New Hampshire

Paige McCarthy, BSN, RN
Clinical RN
University of New Hampshire
Somersworth, New Hampshire

Elise Miles, BSN, RN
Salem, New Hampshire

Amy Morang, MS, APRN, FNP-C
Dartmouth-Hitchcock
  Gastroenterology and Hepatology
Manchester, New Hampshire

Margaret Moriarty-Litz, MS, RN, CNE
Assistant Dean, Undergraduate
  Nursing
Southern New Hampshire
  University
Manchester, New Hampshire

Anastasia Pappas, MS, RN, CNL
Registered Nurse
Lawrence General Hospital
Lawrence, Massachusetts

Lore M. Steinmann, RN, MS, CNL
Charge Nurse
Ledgewood Rehabilitation and
  Skilled Nursing Center
Beverly, Massachusetts

Joan Catherine Widmer, RN, CEN, ASN, BA, MS
Clinical RN
Catholic Medical Center
Manchester, New Hampshire

CONTRIBUTORS TO FIRST EDITION

Sandra Butterfield, RN, BSN
House Supervisor
Prime Healthcare
Chula Vista, California

Terry Capuano, RN, MSN, MBA, FACHE
Chief Operating Officer
Lehigh Valley Health Network
Allentown, Pennsylvania

Margaret Estee, RN
Nurse Manager, Post-Anesthesia
    Care Unit
Maine Medical Center
Portland, Maine

Lynn Geoffrion, RN, MS
Hillsboro, New Hampshire

Tara Herman, RN, BSN
Nurse Manager
Maine Medical Center
Portland, Maine

Deborah Johnson, BSN, RN
Clinical Educator
Tufts Medical Center
Boston, Massachusetts

Lea Ayers La Fave, PhD, RN
Senior Project Director
Community Health Institute/JSI
Bow, New Hampshire

Claire Lindberg, PhD, RN, APN
Professor, School of Nursing,
    Health, and Exercise Science
The College of New Jersey
Ewing, New Jersey

**Anne Marie Logan, RN, MHSA, BSN,
    RAC-CT**
RAI/MDS Coordinator
Durham Veterans Affairs Medical
    Center
Durham, North Carolina

Jeanne A. McLaughlin, MSN, MSEd
President/Chief Executive Officer
Visiting Nurse Association &
    Hospice of VT & NH
West Lebanon, New Hampshire

Patricia Ann Morgan, PhD, RN, CNE
Associate Chair/Assistant Professor
Department of Nursing, University
    of New England
Portland, Maine

Larry Plant, PMH-NP, BC, DNP(c)
Psychiatric Nurse Practitioner
Mercy Hospital
Portland, Maine

Judy Ringer
Author, *Unlikely Teachers: Finding
    the Hidden Gifts in Daily Conflict*
Owner, Power & Presence Training
Portsmouth, New Hampshire

Kathleen Thies, PhD, RN
Senior Nurse Researcher
Elliot Health System
Manchester, New Hampshire

Denise Timberlake, RN, BSN, CNOR
Surgical Services Nurse Manager
St. Mary's Regional Medical Center
Lewiston, Maine

Diane D. Vachon, RN, OCN
Clinical Nurse III, Unit-Based
    Educator
Maine Medical Center
Portland, Maine

Kathleen Welsh, RN, BSN
Senior Product Manager
Haverhill, Massachusetts
Contributors

REVIEWERS

Magdeline Aagard,
  RN, BSN, MBA, EdD
Associate Professor
Department of Nursing
Augsburg College
Minneapolis, Minnesota

Ingrid Brudenell, PhD, RN
Professor
Boise State University
Boise, Idaho

Rosanne J. Curtis, RN, MN, EdD
Dean of Nursing
Mount St. Mary's College
Los Angeles, California

Maria de los Santos, MSN, MPH, ARNP
Clinical Assistant Professor
College of Nursing and Health
  Services
Florida International University
Miami, Florida

Ann Galloway, RN, MS, ACNP/FNP-C
Assistant Professor
Colorado State University–Pueblo
Pueblo, Colorado

Masoud Ghaffari, PhD, MSN/RN,
  MEd(CHE), MT(ASCP), CMA
Associate Professor
College of Nursing
East Tennessee State University
Kingsport, Tennessee

Peggy L. Hawkins, PhD, RN, BC, CNE
Professor of Nursing
College of Saint Mary
Omaha, Nebraska

Nancy Kramer, EdD, MSN, ARNP
Dean
School of Nursing
Allen College
Waterloo, Iowa

Ramona Browder Lazenby,
  EdD, RN, FNP-BC, CNE
Professor
Associate Dean of Nursing
Auburn Montgomery School of
  Nursing
Montgomery, Alabama

Mary Sue Marz, PhD, RN
Professor
School of Nursing
Eastern Michigan University
Ypsilanti, Michigan

Joan C. Masters, EdD, RN
Associate Professor of Nursing
Bellarmine University
Louisville, Kentucky

Antoinette Navalta Herrera,
  EdD(c), MSN, RN
Assistant Professor
California State University–
  Sacramento
Sacramento, California

Joyce Perkins,
  PhD, MS, MA, AHN-BC
Assistant Professor
Augsburg College
Minneapolis, Minnesota

Judith Lloyd Storfjell, PhD, RN
Associate Dean
University of Illinois at Chicago
Executive Director
Institute for Healthcare Innovation
Chicago, Illinois

Connie Vance, EdD, MSN, RN, FAAN
Professor
School of Nursing
The College of New Rochelle
New Rochelle, New York

Daniel Weberg, MHI, BSN, RN, CEN
Director, Academy for Continuing
   Education
Faculty Associate, Masters of
   Healthcare Innovation Program
College of Nursing and Health
   Innovation
Arizona State University
Phoenix, Arizona

John J. Whitcomb, PhD, RN, CCRN
Assistant Professor
Clemson University
Clemson, South Carolina

Lindsey Wilkins, MSN, ARNP
Clinical Assistant Professor
College of Nursing and Health
   Sciences
Florida International University
Miami, Florida

**Kendra Williams-Perez,
   EdD, MSN, CNE**
Assistant Dean of Undergraduate
   Nursing
Professor
Allen College
Cedar Falls, Iowa

Meg Wilson, PhD, RN
Professor
University of Saint Francis
Fort Wayne, Indiana

ABOUT THE AUTHOR

Diana Crowell, PhD, RN, NEA, BC, received her BSN from American International College, her MEd in Counseling from Springfield College, and her MSN in Nursing Management from Anna Maria College. Dr. Crowell received her Doctorate in Leadership in Health Care Systems from Union Institute and University. ANA board certified as Nurse Executive Advanced, her administrative experience ranges from unit supervision to CNO. She has served on faculties of nursing teaching leadership and health policy and as a department director. Dr Crowell has consulted and presented on many aspects of personal and professional leadership. She has been an ANCC Magnet Hospital Recognition Program appraiser and is a member and chapter past president of Sigma Theta Tau International.

ACKNOWLEDGMENTS

Thank you to Joanne DaCunha for seeing my vision for a nursing leadership book based on complexity and for seeking out the interest in a revision and then initiating the project. I appreciate all who contributed case studies based on their rich professional experience and all the students who taught me so much as I taught them in courses using this textbook. And an ongoing thanks to my husband Glen for his constant support, no matter what my projects or professional endeavors have required.

TABLE OF CONTENTS

Complexity Science Concepts and Heath-Care Organizations

1

THE COMPLEXITY LEADERSHIP MODEL

The complexity leader is in the midst of the action; cultivating relationships; accepting feedback; tolerating messy, uncertain situations; and seeking diverse opinions, all while staying centered and self-reflective.

■ OBJECTIVES

- Describe this book's Complexity Leadership Model and its components.
- Discuss the relationships between the components in the model and their impact on leadership.
- Assess your own knowledge of complexity, leadership style, and personal being and awareness.
- Articulate the relationship between complexity leadership and graduate nursing education.

INTRODUCTION

In today's health-care environment, **Complexity Leadership** is not just a new way to lead, but also a new way of thinking that is radically different from the linear, top-down, command-and-control approach that many have experienced in health care and other organizations. Complexity Leadership is based on complexity science theory and takes a new view of health-care organizations as complex adaptive systems.

The concepts of complexity science inform a new worldview of organizations and leadership that is nonlinear, dynamic, often uncertain, and very much relationship-based. A major premise of Complexity Leadership is that putting structures in place in a top-down, command-and-control manner does not necessarily lead to effective outcomes or change people's behavior. In fact, the reverse is often true. Complexity leadership holds that people in relationships throughout an organization, coming together from diverse disciplines and mental models, will create the best structures for moving the organization toward transformation. Because nursing practice is largely relationship-based, many nurses seem to understand this intuitively.

THE COMPLEXITY LEADERSHIP MODEL

The *Complexity Leadership model* presented in this book provides a framework for complexity nursing leadership and is based on concepts from complexity science. It reflects a three-part emphasis on knowledge, leadership style, and personal being and awareness (Fig. 1-1).

The leader's *knowledge* of complexity science concepts and their application to organizations promotes and informs leadership style and personal being and awareness. Together, these components result in the fourth component of the model: actions that can best benefit the organization as a whole and the people within it.

In Complexity Leadership, the *style* is transformational, self-reflective, collaborative, and relationship-based. This is the style that exemplifies complexity. Once the organization is viewed from a complexity perspective, the leader can no longer act in a linear, top-down, authoritarian manner and becomes congruent with complexity principles.

Figure 1-1 *The Complexity Leadership Model.* Knowledge underlies and influences leadership style and personal being and awareness, which in turn yield actions that affect the complex adaptive system.

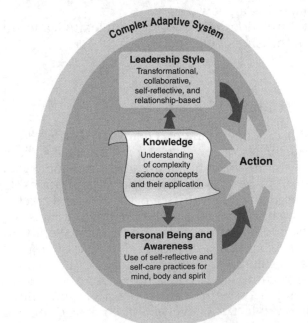

Complex Adaptive System

Leadership Style
Transformational,
collaborative,
self-reflective, and
relationship-based

Knowledge
Understanding
of complexity
science concepts
and their application

Action

Personal Being and Awareness
Use of self-reflective and
self-care practices for
mind, body and spirit

The *personal being and awareness* component includes the use of self-reflective and self-care practices for mind, body, and spiritual health that support and sustain a Complexity Leadership style and effective leadership action. Distancing oneself from linear leadership and adhering to complexity leadership can require personal strength and courage that is best sustained by continuing personal development and self-care practices.

In the fourth component of the model, the complexity leader takes *actions* that employ effective tools and interventions for positive outcomes, growth, and change. The actions taken by the complexity leader are the natural extension of and congruent with complexity science.

Each of this book's three units addresses the major components of the Complexity Leadership Model and the science that underlies it. In each chapter, special features, such as case studies, self-assessments, self-reflective questions, and critical thinking exercises, are provided to help apply complexity leadership concepts to nursing and to health-care organizational leadership.

COMPLEXITY SCIENCE AND LEADERSHIP

The key force behind the Complexity Leadership Model is knowledge of complexity science theory and concepts, and an understanding of how these concepts relate to seeing health-care organizations and systems as complex adaptive systems. Indeed, complexity science theory is the study of complex adaptive systems. It considers the pattern of relationships in the system, how they are sustained, how they self-regulate and self-organize, and how outcomes emerge. It includes the input of quantitative and qualitative data. It teaches that everything is related or connected at some level and that systems thrive on relationships and their intersections rather than on control of all aspects of the process.

Once thinking changes from a linear view to one of complexity, the shift is paradigmatic. One's knowledge and understanding of complexity influences one's leadership style. The cognitive shift that occurs when organizations and leadership are viewed through a complexity lens (Lindberg, Zimmerman, and Plsek, 2001) calls forth a transformational, collaborative, reflective, relationship-based leadership style.

This complexity leadership style is best supported by a personal being and awareness that employs self-reflective, self-care practices for mind, body, and spiritual health. The focus on personal development presented in this book is unique and is included because it is difficult to maintain a complexity leadership style without developing and sustaining key personal qualities and practices.

The Complexity Leadership Model assumes a high level of congruence between and among the components. In other words, leaders with knowledge of complex adaptive systems have a complexity view that, in turn, requires a leadership style congruent with the precepts of the complex adaptive system approach. This, in turn, calls for a full awareness of one's personal reactions, emotions, prejudices, tendencies, impact on others, and ability to cope and relate in a very demanding role. A complexity leader is in the midst of the action, cultivating relationships, accepting feedback, tolerating uncertain situations, seeking diverse opinions, listening to multiple views, and as much as possible remaining calm and centered. Mindell (1995) calls this approach *sitting in the fire.*

With linear leadership in a top-down organization, leaders may consider themselves to be outside the system and feel protected and less vulnerable. The complexity leader, who is naturally more vulnerable because there is so much focus on relationships, needs to develop personal aspects of leadership.

There are health-care leaders who are intellectually fascinated with complexity science theory but do not see how commitment to the science requires either a transformational leadership style congruent with complexity science or a willingness to grow and transform oneself in order to practice transformational leadership. For example, someone may subscribe to a complexity view of organizations that entails complex relationships, surprise, and unpredictability. But if that same person tends to an authoritarian style of leadership that is not in keeping with complexity, the individual will be less effective.

Of even more personal difficulty for a leader is to attempt a complexity leadership style without the emotional and social makeup to support it. This can be extremely stressful personally and to others. For instance, if a leader who believes in people self-organizing and in decentralized decision making is personally more comfortable with tight control, that leader cannot be effective or centered without first recognizing that preference and then working to change it. An assumption of complexity leadership is that it is possible to change through self-awareness and personal self-reflective practices.

Everyone has unique behavioral tendencies, personalities, and approaches to life. The Complexity Leadership Model assumes that one can learn through education and self-reflective practices to develop the behaviors that support becoming a complexity leader. The complexity leader's approach is based on complexity thinking long before any action is taken. For an example, see *A Case for Complexity,* which describes Helen Restin, whose thinking and approach to her new chief nursing officer position exemplifies complexity leadership.

THINKING LIKE A COMPLEXITY LEADER

Helen thinks like a complexity leader. She long ago discarded linear, top-down thinking and views her organization as a complex adaptive system that can self-organize with the right leadership. Complexity

A CASE FOR COMPLEXITY

Helen Restin was getting ready for work on the Monday of her second week in her new position as chief nursing officer (CNO) at City South Medical Center (CSMC). CSMC had been formed by a merger between City Medical Center (CMC) and Southside Hospital (SSH). Much of the process of moving services and integrating staff has been scheduled to occur during the upcoming year, in a series of 3-month periods. The decision to merge the two hospitals was made by the board about a year ago. The last 6 months have seen some personnel changes (one being the new CNO) and work with the community to gain acceptance and support as well as preliminary facility planning.

The chief executive officer (CEO) of the merged organization, Jim Jason, had been the CEO of CMC for 3 years. The previous CNO did not share Jim's comfort with and enthusiasm for the uncertainty that accompanies a merger, so she left for another position. She preferred more order and less change in her work life. As for SSH, both the CEO and CNO decided to retire after long and successful careers building SSH into a respected institution. In fact, they had been instrumental in fostering the merger as the next best step for the community. The retiring CNO left SSH a well-developed, professional, and self-governed nursing organization. In contrast, the CMC nurses did not operate on a self-governance model, but recently they had been bringing the idea forward to their leadership.

The medical staff shared many of the community patients and so viewed the merger as positive. They welcomed the opportunity to operate with one set of policies, procedures, and expectations. The chief of the medical staff, Stan Whaley, was on the CNO search team and was very supportive of Helen's selection. Helen was expected to be a strong leader in this merger implementation. She was chosen because of the experience she gained in her two previous positions. In the first, she took part in a similar merger at the director level. Then, as CNO of a midsized hospital, she had spearheaded a successful Magnet Recognition Program application. Becoming CNO brought Helen back to the region where she grew up and seemed like the right challenge for her.

During graduate school, Helen studied complexity science and complex adaptive systems and how those concepts can be applied to health-care organizations. She found this knowledge very helpful in her pursuit of Magnet designation in her previous position, and she came to understand that linear leadership is not very compatible with a Magnet paradigm of structured empowerment, self-governance, and an expectation of innovation. With Helen's knowledge of how complex adaptive systems work, she knew to expect surprise, accept uncertainty, and value and appreciate diversity.

Continued

A CASE FOR COMPLEXITY—cont'd

At SSMC, she found two cultures merging with diverse disciplines and mental models as well as different expectations of leaders. Relationships were crucial, and she knew she would not have complete control of the people or the system. She realized that complicated rules, policies, and procedures imposed from the top down would not work in the long run to effect a successful merger. Helen's intent was to create an environment to foster relationships so that people across the organization could come together to create the most effective structures.

Although Helen's leadership style was participative and relationship-centered, (a complexity leadership approach), she had developed some personal awareness about how others might perceive her. She was such an upbeat person and open to new ideas and related so well to people that she occasionally let her enthusiasm interfere with really listening to others and allowing time for their ideas to emerge. Through self-reflection and self-care practices, she had learned to recognize the signals and to slow down, breathe, and give others space and time.

Helen had been asked to take 3 months to assess the overall situation and to develop a plan for implementing the merger from a patient care perspective. She saw the facilities' logistics and bringing together two disparate nursing departments as great challenges. But her immediate action was to connect with others and to build relationships throughout the organizations because she believed that plans would never work if they were hers alone, without ideas that were widely solicited and shared. She really was a champion of distributed leadership and referred to her approach as "relate, relate, relate, and listen, listen, listen." She would put the start of a plan in place once she knew the players and how things currently worked. Helen was eager to begin this exciting new leadership adventure.

science and complex adaptive systems are described in more detail in Chapters 2 and 3. Chapter 4 presents actual research and practice models developed and implemented by nursing leaders who embrace complexity and base their work on these concepts.

A good way to prepare for the material in these chapters is with a little self-assessment. Do you *think* like a complexity leader? The following complexity leadership quiz can help you assess your thinking about organizations and how close to complexity thinking you are at this time. The quiz can generate some fruitful discussion as well.

For each question, choose the one answer in each situation that you think is the closest to complexity thinking. The correct answers appear at the end of the chapter, and explanations are given in later chapters.

1. *When events do not turn out as expected, I think:*
   a. the planning was not thorough enough.
   b. the person or group responsible should be identified.
   c. a review of the system is needed.
   d. there may be opportunity in this happening.
2. *When strategic planning is required, I think:*
   a. each step needs to be spelled out clearly.
   b. the complexity of the plan should equal the complexity of the expected results.
   c. there may not be a correlation between details and results.
   d. experts should be employed to develop the plans.
3. *With regard to organizational-wide planning for system change, I think:*
   a. changing the reporting structure encourages people to change.
   b. the larger one's span of control, the harder it is to effect change.
   c. people in effective relationships can produce effective system-wide change.
   d. informing people in detail about the change will help them to accept it.
4. *With regard to the most effective dissemination of information, I think:*
   a. sending out information along formal reporting lines ensures dissemination.
   b. information should be shared on a need-to-know basis to reduce rumors.
   c. choosing one information-sharing vehicle, such as a newsletter, fosters information transfer.
   d. multiple methods and the free flow of information will reach nearly everyone.
5. *Visibility of senior management:*
   a. is best accomplished by specific meetings at specific times to instill trust.
   b. is best done through connections with middle management.
   c. is accomplished in multiple ways of relating and communicating across the organization.
   d. is not expected by most people because they know how busy senior managers are.
6. *The following is true about best-run team and staff meetings:*
   a. tight control with a firm pre-published agenda gets things done.
   b. a loose and free-wheeling approach gives everyone a chance to be creative and caring.
   c. there is a correlation between the duration of the meeting and the quality of the results.
   d. a well-organized agenda with time for new ideas to emerge is effective.

7. *Rumors and negative conversations are best handled by:*
   a. insisting on positive, upbeat conversations and discussions.
   b. keeping the correct positive information in circulation.
   c. seeking information and feedback.
   d. ignoring them unless they become destructive.

ACTING LIKE A COMPLEXITY LEADER

Chapters 5 through 8 focus on leadership—the history, styles, actions, and contemporary models that reflect aspects of complexity leadership. In preparation for this material, try a little more self-assessment. Do you *act* like a complexity leader? The following quiz will help you assess what actions you would take and how close they are to the way a complexity leader would proceed in a given situation. No answers are wrong, but one answer is closest to complexity leadership behavior in each situation. Correct answers appear at the end of the chapter, and full discussions appear in the chapters to come.

1. *When contemplating a need for change in a system, structure, or process, I would:*
   a. gather a small group of the most knowledgeable people to draft a plan.
   b. assign a special project manager to develop the plan.
   c. confer with peers in other organizations to adopt their proven initiative.
   d. cast a wide net for idea and practices.
2. *When forming a task force or work group, I would:*
   a. select from the senior leadership group.
   b. make sure the power players are in the room.
   c. select people with diverse mental models and views.
   d. look for compatibility of personality and work styles.
3. *As director of critical care and the emergency department, I hear that nurses in the emergency department are complaining about changes in admitting procedures. My most likely approach would be to:*
   a. ask their unit manager to settle them down.
   b. go to the next staff meeting and ask for feedback.
   c. ask staff development to re-educate them on the procedure.
   d. circulate to observe and be open to hearing how things are going.
4. *To create the climate for more nurses to become involved in self-governance committees, I would:*
   a. make sure it is included in the RN job description.
   b. hold a meeting to encourage participation.
   c. make sure that the achievements of the nurses already involved are recognized and rewarded.
   d. connect it to salary.

5. *Patient satisfaction scores for nurses' caring and listening have dropped for three quarters in a row. I most likely would:*
   a. ignore it because the staff has been very stressed lately.
   b. ask staff development to hold some classes.
   c. determine which nurses specifically are responsible.
   d. disseminate the concern widely and seek ideas for improvement.

6. *The outpatient clinic staff has fashioned its own way to process admissions.Although it seems to be easier and more comfortable for patients, the procedure does not adhere to established protocol. I would most likely first:*
   a. ask staff development to re-educate them on the proper protocol.
   b. leave them alone because it works for them.
   c. make a visit and ask them to describe their process.
   d. ask the unit manager to correct the situation.

7. *Because of new regional health insurance regulations and a shift in the community's population, there is considerable uncertainty and dis- agreement among administrative, medical, and clinical staff and finance whether to expand some services. As a complexity leader, my approach would be to:*
   a. see what other health-care organizations have done under these circumstances.
   b. bring all parties together to share ideas.
   c. encourage senior leadership to decide based on available information.
   d. do nothing until more is known.

ASSESSING PERSONAL DEVELOPMENT

Personal development is an important facet of effective leadership and is discussed in Chapters 9 through 12. Developing certain personal traits and practices can prepare leaders to meet the demands of Complexity Leadership. This chapter has already shown that self-assessment and willingness to grow are integral to Complexity Leadership. To take this concept further, try the two accompanying tools for assessing your self awareness (Box 1–1) and your level of self-care practices (Box 1–2). As before, there are no wrong answers. This is a values clarification method to start you on your own complexity leadership journey.

CONTEMPORARY NURSING LEADERSHIP EXPECTATIONS

The Complexity Leadership Model—indeed, complexity leadership itself—is useful for advanced practice nurses who occupy both formal and informal leadership positions. Advanced practice nurses not in

Box 1–1	SELF-ASSESSMENT

PERSONAL BEING AND SELF-AWARENESS
Assess your behavioral tendencies and emotional reactions on a scale of 1 to 10 (with 1 being less and 10 being more).

Need for control	1 2 3 4 5 6 7 8 9 10
Need for order	1 2 3 4 5 6 7 8 9 10
Need for certainty	1 2 3 4 5 6 7 8 9 10
Handling surprise	1 2 3 4 5 6 7 8 9 10
Seeking feedback	1 2 3 4 5 6 7 8 9 10
Handling feedback	1 2 3 4 5 6 7 8 9 10
Being present	1 2 3 4 5 6 7 8 9 10
Fully listening	1 2 3 4 5 6 7 8 9 10
Staying centered	1 2 3 4 5 6 7 8 9 10
Aware of feelings	1 2 3 4 5 6 7 8 9 10

Self-reflection
What have I learned about myself?

Box 1–2	SELF-ASSESSMENT

SELF-CARE PRACTICES
Assess your level of attention to the following self-care practices on a scale of 1 to 10 (with 1 being less and 10 being more).

Exercise	1 2 3 4 5 6 7 8 9 10
Healthy eating	1 2 3 4 5 6 7 8 9 10
Medical care	1 2 3 4 5 6 7 8 9 10
Safety (seat belts, etc.)	1 2 3 4 5 6 7 8 9 10
Time management	1 2 3 4 5 6 7 8 9 10
Spiritual practice	1 2 3 4 5 6 7 8 9 10
Family relationships	1 2 3 4 5 6 7 8 9 10
Social relationships	1 2 3 4 5 6 7 8 9 10
Work/life balance	1 2 3 4 5 6 7 8 9 10
Clarity of values	1 2 3 4 5 6 7 8 9 10

Self-reflection
What have I learned about myself?

formal leadership positions often are called upon to be leaders in their organizations. In multidisciplinary settings, it is the nurse who is the constant presence. Coupled with their organizational skills, nurses are expected to solve problems, develop new programs, and in general are the glue that keeps things together and systems functioning.

Such a challenge calls for an understanding of organizational systems, effective leadership styles, and personal development to cope with the demands of leadership.

When nurses move into leadership roles, from practice to management, many experience culture shock and some cognitive dissonance if they enter a senior management environment that is linear, quantitative, and command-and-control, with little emphasis on relationships.

The Complexity Leadership Model and the material presented in this book are fully applicable to the reality of nursing leadership. For those already in leadership roles, it can enhance and enrich their current practice, giving them a broader view of their organizations as well as tools and interventions to support their leadership. This is not a nursing administration text with a focus on budgets and human resources practice. It is excellent preparation for roles such as clinical nurse specialist (CNS), clinical nurse leader (CNL), nurse practitioner (NP), or doctor of nursing practice (DNP).

Nurse executives will find this text valuable as they strive to bring their nursing leadership team toward a complexity perspective. They can then be in a better position to influence their colleagues in other disciplines and departments to embrace complexity behaviors and promote distributed leadership.

The Institute of Medicine (2004) determined that the following evidenced-based management components are essential for effective leadership in health-care organizations:

- Balancing the tension between production efficiency and reliability
- Creating and sustaining trust throughout the organization
- Actively managing the process of change
- Involving workers in decision making pertaining to work design and work flow
- Using knowledge management practices to establish "learning organizations"

All of the above components are illustrative of aspects of complexity leadership. The ANCC Magnet Recognition Program (2008) evaluates nursing within hospital and health-care agency settings based on ANCC's Forces of Magnetism. The quality of the nursing leadership is paramount in creating an environment of structured empowerment. In this environment, nurses can enact professional practice with autonomy and the respect of the health-care community. A Magnet CNO exemplifies transformational, relationship-based complexity leadership traits. The Magnet Model is discussed in Chapter 6.

The American Organization of Nurse Executives (AONE) sees the competencies of communication and relationship building, leadership, knowledge of health-care systems, plus professionalism and business skills to be necessary for effective fulfillment of the leadership role (IOM, 2010). These qualities and competencies are reflective of all graduate nursing education and certainly exemplify the roles of CNL and DNP.

Nursing Graduate-Level Education

The American Association of Colleges of Nursing (AACN) *Essentials of Master's Education in Nursing* delineates expectations for competencies and serves as guidelines for curriculum development. Essential II: Organizational and Systems Leadership directly relates to the content in this text. The competencies in this Essential include the use of complexity science and systems theory in leadership to implement change and new designs for delivery of best-quality health care. Effective communication within the interdisciplinary team is most elemental. Successful leadership entails grasping how the health-care delivery systems are organized, including legal, economic, and political factors.

The CNL competencies build upon Essential II to emphasize collaboration, systems theory, an understanding of how systems work, and taking on the role of leader within an interdisciplinary team (AACN, 2013). The DNP uses the *Essentials* as a foundation as well to enhance and enrich previous learning and achieve this terminal degree. It is expected that the standard for a nurse executive will go beyond the master's degree to the level of DNP. McCaffrey (2012) expresses the importance of understanding systems, systems change, and complex adaptive systems in her text describing the DNP role.

SUMMARY

As the health-care system evolves, advanced practice nurses will be expected to be trailblazers and fully contemporary contributors to the system. Complexity leadership will prepare nurses to assume this very important role. Begun and White (2008, p. 256) describe a complexity-inspired approach to leadership as one that "recognizes that the future is unknowable and unpredictable but that its emerging features are shaped by those individuals and organizations with the competencies to explore, connect and make sense."

This introductory chapter provides an overview of the Complexity Leadership model and an opportunity to assess one's complexity thinking, leadership style, and personal development. Chapter 2 reviews the relevant history of complexity science and concepts, which serve as the foundational knowledge of complex adaptive systems and health-care organizations. This is knowledge essential to complexity thinking and leadership.

1–1 CRITICAL THINKING EXERCISE ■■■■■

Look back at the questions and answers for the Complexity Leadership Quiz. Choose one group of questions, and use the *Case for Complexity* to describe how Helen Restin exemplifies these complexity concepts in her leadership thinking and actions with examples.

QUESTIONS FOR SELF-REFLECTION ■■■■■

1. Imagine you are Helen Restin. How would you plan your second week? Who would you meet? What formal events might you hold? What would you consider early priorities for building relationships? What information is essential to know as soon as possible?
2. Can you recall being in a situation in which you could see what was happening within your organization but did not know how to act in the leadership role in that situation?
3. Have you been in a situation in which you knew how to act as a leader but found it very difficult or stressful to act as you believed you should because of your emotional response?

Self-Reflection: What Have I Learned?

_____

_____

_____

_____

_____

_____

_____

_____

_____

ANSWERS TO KNOWLEDGE AND ACTION QUIZZES
Knowledge Quiz: 1d, 2c, 3c, 4d, 5c, 6d, 7c
Action Quiz: 1d, 2c, 3d, 4c, 5d, 6c, 7b

CES

American Association of Colleges of Nursing. (2007). *White paper on the role of the clinical nurse leader.* Retrieved April 8, 2010, from http://www.aacn.nche.edu/publications/whitepapers/clinicalnurseleader.htm

American Association of Colleges of Nursing. (2013). *Competencies and curricular expectations for clinical nurse leader education and practice.* Retrieved March 5, 2015, from http://www.aacn.nche.edu/cnl/CNL-Competencies-October-2013.pdf

American Nurses Credentialing Center. (2008). *Application manual: Magnet recognition program.* Silver Spring, MD: Author.

Begun, J., & White, K. (2008) The challenge of change: Inspiring leadership. In C. Lindberg, S. Nash, & C. Lindberg (eds.). *On the edge: Nursing in the age of complexity.* Bordentown, NJ: PlexusPress.

Institute of Medicine of the National Academies. (2004). *Keeping patients safe: Transforming the work environment of nurses.* Washington, D.C.: The National Academies Press.

Lindberg, C., Zimmerman, B., & Plsek, P. (2001). *Edgeware: Complexity resources for health care leaders.* Bordentown, NJ: Plexus Institute. Retrieved April 8, 2010, from http://www.plexusinstitute.org/edgeware/archive/think/

McCaffrey, R, (2012). *Doctor of nursing practice: Enhancing professional development.* Philadelphia, PA: F.A. Davis Company.

Mindell, A. (1995). *Sitting in the fire: Large group transformation using conflict and diversity.* Portland, OR: Lao Tse Press.

16 **Complexity Leadership** | *Nursing's Role in Health-Care Delivery*

2

MAJOR CONCEPTS OF COMPLEXITY SCIENCE THEORY

The complexity leader sees organizations as living systems composed of people in relationship, not as machines with gears, levers, and clockwork precision.

■ OBJECTIVES

- Discuss the historical development of complexity science.
- Define major concepts of complexity science.
- Apply complexity science concepts to organizational situations.
- Compare and contrast linear and complexity thinking.

INTRODUCTION

This chapter tells the history of science as it relates to an understanding of complexity science. Specific concepts of complexity science are defined, explored, and connected to new ways of viewing human systems and organizations. Chapters 2 and 3 explain the theoretical foundation of the Complexity Leadership Model. It is essential for leaders to understand this foundation and to integrate it into their thinking so it can influence leadership styles and actions in a meaningful way. Although foundational material can sometimes seem esoteric and abstract, the goal of these chapters is to present the material so that, with some attention and self-reflection, these new science concepts can become real and accessible.

The history of science presented here begins with the medieval view, which was spiritual and organic, and moves on to the Age of Enlightenment, where the approach changed to quantification. As biology developed and began to compete with the idea that everything was mechanical, the shift toward whole systems began. The new science of quantum physics was presenting the notion of worlds unseen yet connected. We trace the history of complexity science from chaos theory, with its butterfly effect, attractors, and fractals, to self-organizing systems and on to complex adaptive systems applied to living organizations.

An understanding of how this science developed and influenced management and leadership theorists is important in becoming a complexity leader. Additionally, it can help explain the apparent disorder and difficulty that is part of the work life in organizations. The ability to not only understand but use the language of complexity is essential to complexity thinking and to becoming a complexity leader.

Complexity leadership is based on new ways of explaining organizations. This new systems approach to leadership is derived from the study of complex living systems, a distinct contrast from a mechanistic view of the world. For decades, the paradigm of scientific management and classical management theory became so ingrained that most managers think in terms of formal structures linked by clear lines as the path to coordination, command, and control (Capra, 2002). The journey from a tight "plan, organize, control, and direct" style of management to complexity leadership mirrors the history of science since medieval times.

Just as there can be tension between old and new management approaches, there is historical scientific tension between the parts and the whole, the mechanistic and the organic, reductionistic thinking and systems thinking. Biologists came to understand that matter (structure, quantity, substance) and form (pattern, order, quality) were both necessary for development and evolution in biological processes. Knowing about the building blocks of an organism without understanding its patterns and processes is incomplete. This is the tension between the parts and the whole (Capra, 2002).

EVENTS TO CONSIDER FROM A COMPLEXITY PERSPECTIVE

Consider how the following world and organizational events might be explained. First, in 1989, the Berlin Wall, which had remained in place so rigidly since World War II, fell. How did that happen without a strategic plan, a CEO, or long-range planning?

Second, the CEO of a large hospital system decrees that a large-scale organizational change will take place. After a flurry of activity, task forces, plans, and projects, months to years later little difference can be seen in how the organization operates or that the change has taken hold or that any outcomes are evident.

Third, one person or a very small group, typically at a local or lower level, expresses an idea or starts a practice that spreads throughout the organization, usually not through formal channels, and that results in a widespread change in behavior.

All three of these examples can be explained when one's view shifts from a mechanistic, linear explanation of how society and organizations work in reality to a complexity whole-systems perspective. This shift in view requires, first, a shift in paradigmatic thinking and, second, a new language. Reflect on these situations as you read. There are discussion questions and explanation at the end of the chapter.

HISTORICAL PERSPECTIVE

Historically, the medieval view was one of an organic, living, spiritual universe. Discoveries during the Age of Enlightenment by Newton, Galileo, Copernicus, and Descartes launched the Scientific Revolution. Measurement and quantification replaced qualitative ways of exploring phenomena. René Descartes viewed nature as divided between mind and matter. The material world could be analyzed by breaking things into their smallest parts; this has been termed a reductionist approach. These scientists conceptualized the world as a perfect machine, measured by mathematics, thus refuting the earlier spiritually based philosophy.

Biochemistry's chemical processes had not yet been discovered. As scientists gradually understood biological processes, there were swings between reducing everything to the parts in the cells to looking at patterns, relationships, and processes of self-organization. The seeds of systems thinking started to emerge as well as the idea of organized complexity. In other words, a whole cannot be understood by examining its parts in isolation; it requires the context of other wholes. Quantum theory revealed that there are no hard and solid material properties at the subatomic level, but only patterns, connections, and probabilities. Systems can be thought of as interconnecting networks or a web. The systems approach is all about connections, the whole in context giving meaning to the parts, not the other way around (Capra, 2002).

Nursing theorist Martha Rogers (1970) based her work, *The Science of Unitary Human Beings,* on new science quantum theory. At the time, her theory was considered rather esoteric and not very relevant to the practical aspects of nursing practice and health care. Rogers proposed a systems-connected view of nursing science before these concepts were fully developed and articulated. There is now a more complete and accessible complexity science language. Margaret Newman's *Health as Expanding Consciousness* (1994) and Jean Watson's *Nursing: The Philosophy and Science of Caring* (1979/2008) draw from the new science concepts to further explain and apply nursing in a postmodern world.

Margaret Wheatley's book, *Leadership and the New Science,* (2006) delivered these concepts to management and leadership. She brought science and leadership together in a startling and accessible manner that spread rapidly through the organizational management and leadership community. Wheatley writes in her introduction: "Each of us lives and works in organizations designed from Newtonian images of the universe. We manage by separating things into parts. We believe that influence occurs as a direct result of force exerted from one person to another. We engage in complex planning for a world that we keep expecting to be predictable and search continually for better methods of measuring and perceiving the world" (p. 7).

Complexity science is the term given to a collection of scientific ideas and studies derived from, among others, quantum physics, chaos theory, and systems theory. Table 2–1 reviews some of the key concepts in this way of thinking. Members of no one discipline are involved; rather, many. These include biologists, physicists, anthropologists, economists, sociologists, leadership and management scholars and, of great importance, nursing theorists (Lindberg, Zimmerman, and Plsek, 2001). Systems thinking went from studying the parts to know the whole to the view that the whole can be

(text continues on page 23)

Table 2–1 COMPLEXITY SCIENCE KEY CONCEPTS

The following are key terms, definitions, and examples of some major complexity concepts as they relate to organizational life.

TERM	DEFINITION	EXAMPLES
Attractors	• Points of attraction Used to describe the overall behavior of a complex system in which patterns of energy attract more energy • Three types: point, periodic, and strange attractors	• *Point attractors:* All pulling together in a crisis, one great idea, or a transformational charismatic leader • *Periodic attractors:* Joint Commission preparation and visit • *Strange attractors:* Irregular and random-appearing organizational culture
Butterfly effect	• A small unintended event that produces enormous effects with positive or negative consequences because of sensitivity of people and structures to initial conditions	• Just as a butterfly flaps it wings, "flaps" happen in organizations. A casual comment in a meeting flies throughout the organization, creating a huge misunderstanding and enormous energy to correct the misunderstanding (Wheatley, 1995).

Table 2–1	COMPLEXITY SCIENCE KEY CONCEPTS—cont'd	
TERM	**DEFINITION**	**EXAMPLES**
Distributed leadership	• A process that includes accountability and contributions from nurses at all levels	• Shared governance Magnet hospitals create an environment where it is expected that direct-care registered nurses at all levels have decision-making opportunities.
Emergence	• Unexpected new ideas, structures, and patterns (novelty) arising from people in relationship • Creativity and change to a higher order is the natural state of a system.	• Atoms form chemical bonds to become emergent structures called molecules. • Human beings buy, sell, and trade to meet their individual and family needs, thus creating the emergent structure known as the market. • Groups of independent agents in the system cooperate and compete, seeking self-consistency and mutual accommodation to transcend themselves and become more (Waldrop, 1992).
Fractals	• Similar shapes found in nature or generated with computer modeling • Shapes nested within shapes of descending size	• In organizations, systems within systems in descending order of size: organization—division—department—unit • One idea or principle iterated throughout an organization • In health care, a comfort and caring approach enacted in every corner of the organization

Continued

Table 2–1	COMPLEXITY SCIENCE KEY CONCEPTS—cont'd	
TERM	**DEFINITION**	**EXAMPLES**
Independent agents	• In a living system, individuals who act at the local level but affect the whole system • Response to local conditions and personal circumstances	• People in the complex adaptive system are independent and cannot be forced to comply. Leaders can create a system in which individuals are willingly motivated to contribute to the whole in positive ways
Nonlinearity	• Small-change efforts that result in large effects • Large-change efforts producing very little transformation • Often no direct cause and effect • Everything is connected and very sensitive to even tiny perturbations (Waldrop, 1992).	• A nurse in an ambulatory surgery department learns therapeutic touch (TT) and uses it in her practice. Other nurses see the benefits and learn and practice it. A physician sees the positive results among patients and writes orders for TT and tells colleagues, who in turn request TT. The reputation of the service spreads in the community as patients relate how they were cared for. As the reputation spreads, demand for the service grows in thegeographic area. People request their outpatient surgery at that hospital.
Self-organization	• New structure and order that emerges from within the system, not necessarily with a leader giving directions but from the interactive relationships within and at local levels • May have positive or negative results	• In crisis situations, people often pull together, self-organize, and accomplish amazing things. • Mobs can self-organize for less than beneficial outcomes.

Table 2–1	COMPLEXITY SCIENCE KEY CONCEPTS—cont'd	
TERM	**DEFINITION**	**EXAMPLES**
Simple rules	• Simple rules can lead to complex, emergent, innovative system behavior. • Applied to organizations, simple rules provide very effective organizational outcomes.	• In *Crossing The Quality Chasm* (2001), the Institute of Medicine's groundbreaking work for improving health care, the six aims for improvement can be seen as simple rules for an effective health-care system. • Health care should be: Safe, effective, patient-centered, timely, efficient, and equitable.

known in terms of connectedness, relationships, context, and patterns (Capra, 1996).

DEVELOPMENT OF COMPLEXITY SCIENCE

Ludwig von Bertalanffy studied systems between the 1940s and 1960s and produced his seminal work in 1968 on General Systems Theory. He is credited with the first formulation of a comprehensive theoretical framework describing principles of organization in living systems. His work was a catalyst for the shift in paradigm from mechanistic to holistic thinking, such as systems thinking about living systems (Capra, 1996).

Chaos Theory

Chaos theory (also called dynamic systems theory) is one contributor to complexity science and is based in mathematics. Chaos, derived from Greek, means *formless matter.* Chaos has no one definition as it relates to chaos theory. Gleick (1987) provides a representative definition as "the apparently random recurrent behavior in a simple deterministic clock-like system" (p. 306). Chaos theory is about patterns and flow, such as weather or cars traveling and clustering on the highway. Gleick named it a science of the global nature of systems. Chaos concepts became topics for discussion and suggestions for a broader use beyond the laboratory, especially the idea that while a system may look chaotic, confused, and disordered, there is an underlying order present. In a living system, the disorder can be called turbulence, but the edge of the chaos is where change and creative ordering takes place through a dynamic, holistic, and reciprocal process.

The tension between order and chaos is part of the growth process for new order to emerge (Ray, Didominic, Dittman, et al., 1995).

Nonlinearity

Nonlinearity is an essential element in chaos theory. One of the hardest notions for mainstream scientists to accept was that the universe is not a machine-like entity where actions are caused by previous actions in a mechanistic manner (Peat, 1990). In the 1960s and 1970s, meteorologist Edward Lorenz conducted some of the earliest research using computer modeling to predict weather more reliably. To his surprise, Lorenz discovered that a very small change in an equation (input) could result in a very large and unpredictable change in the system. He termed this occurrence *sensitive dependence on initial conditions*. Scientists were seeing that systems in computer models and weather were nonlinear, unpredictable, and full of surprises. The metaphorical anecdote that a butterfly flapping its wings in one part of the world may result in a tornado in another illustrates sensitive dependence on initial conditions and has been called *the butterfly effect*. Lorenz continued his work with computer modeling, programming nonlinear equations to be calculated over and over and plotted randomly. While the plotting was random, the patterns that developed did not look random at all, but were beautiful designs. He named these designs *strange attractors*. Interestingly, early on, one of his strange attractors resembled a butterfly (Gleick, 1987).

Attractors

Attractors shape the patterns of behaviors in complex systems. There are three classifications. First, there are *point attractors,* such as when all activities in a system tend toward a single point. For example, a marble circling a bowl will always find its way to the bottom. Second. there are *periodic attractors,* which occur when behavior is repeated at regular intervals, such as the movement of celestial bodies.Third, *strange attractors* are operative when the system appears to behave randomly with no single point or regularity, but over time, complex patterns can be discerned. Heartbeats and weather systems are examples of strange attractor behavior (Eoyang, 1997).

An example of an attractor not related to computer modeling is an experiment conducted with sand and music. When sand is poured in a random pile upon a drum skin surface and music is played below that surface, the vibrations of the music cause the sand to shift and form a distinct patterned design, chaos transforming into order. Wheatley (1995) describes chaos and order as partners because, as chaos occurs, attractors are the phenomena that pull the system into new order.

Fractals

French mathematician Benoît Mandelbrot was developing fractal geometry in the same period when Lorenz was working, the 1960s and 1970s. Mandelbrot studied the geometry of a wide variety of natural forms, such as shorelines, trees, and leaves, and saw many common features. He coined the term *fractal* to explain the shapes found in nature and generated with computer modeling. These shapes were scaled with characteristic patterns repeating in descending scales, smaller and smaller and with self-similarity. The sub-shape can be identified and is for the most part identical to the overall shape (Gleick, 1987).

Self-Organizing Systems

Scientists, physicists, biologists, mathematicians, and social scientists were bringing together their ideas about systems, and management/ organizational theorists were taking notice. Ilya Prigogine, in his physics of becoming, described systems as continuously importing free energy from the environment and exporting entropy, thus self-organizing into stable structures called *dissipative structures*. These structures have within them the means to renew themselves, a process called *autopoiesis*. Biological systems are autopoietic, self-renewing, as opposed to machines, which are termed *allopoietic*, not able to renew themselves (Jantsch, 1980).

In a self-organizing manner through feedback, self-reference, and information, newer systems are created. Self-reference is the process whereby a biological system refers back to itself for further direction for renewal, to its own genetic code and experience as opposed to a machine, which takes direction from outside itself. Self-renewal in living systems (autopoiesis) happens while integrity of the structure is maintained, and it depends upon self-reference. The human body is a prime example, with DNA as the self-reference point. Jantsch (1980), in referring to autopoiesis and self-renewal, states that "a dissipative structure knows indeed what it has to import and export in order to maintain and renew itself. It needs nothing else but reference to itself" (p. 40). The creation of new systems occurs in the space between the edge of chaos and the new system. At that point, one of maximum instability, there are many possible choices or directions open, which may result in collapse or change and a reordering to a new order or pattern of behavior (Ray, Didominic, Dittman, et al., 1995).

Another aspect of an open, self-organizing system is its relationship with its environment. (see *A Case for Complexity*.) The relationship includes the exchange of matter, energy, and information and being ever open to the new and unexpected (novelty). The system, in order to be in an exchange environment, has an internal state of disequilibrium. Without that internal state, the process would die down. All systems have characteristic patterns, and these patterns are necessary for self-renewal. The processes are multilevel; in other words, there are systems within systems within systems (Jantsch 1980). This embeddedness is also an example of the fractal nature of systems.

A CASE FOR COMPLEXITY

A highly functional intensive care nursery (ICN) in a rural JCAHO-accredited Magnet hospital was an apparently stable system. Nurses on the unit had an average of 12 years in their current positions, and they participated in the operation of the unit through shared governance and quality improvement efforts. Many were involved in the design of a new unit when the hospital changed locations. Over a 10-year period, the unit expanded its capacity from 16 beds to 32 beds. Although most of the nurses worked with one another on this unit for years, the unit lacked the base staff to support the unpredictable staffing needs as the unit expanded. In addition, the rural location of the medical center presented challenges related to recruitment and retention of new nurses.

One controversial solution to meeting staffing needs through the expansion and the nursing shortage included the utilization of travel nurses (TNs). The nurses were aware that the use of TNs is controversial for several reasons. They are expensive, costing the unit more than it costs for staff nurses. In some facilities, when the census is down and staff are called off from working, TNs get the hours because they are paid by contract. In addition, TNs may not be required to float to pediatric or maternity units when additional staffing is needed in those areas. TNs may be contracted for up to 3 to 6 months at each assignment.

A common belief exists that the nursing care provided by TNs is less than optimal because they do not know the work environment as well as employed staff nurses and have not developed strong working relationships with the other nurses and therefore represent a lack of continuity in patient care.

However, the nurses discovered some pros as well. Recent research suggested that there may be benefits to using TNs (or other supplemental nursing staff). TNs working in an ICN are highly skilled specialist clinicians. They bring perspectives that are influenced by working within and across multiple systems. They know what works and have some ideas about why. After considering all these issues, the decision was made to employ TNs.

TNs play a role in quality improvement in this organization because they have knowledge about what works elsewhere. They provide perspective on new equipment, models of care, staffing patterns, and sharing of tips and tricks of patient care. They can "see the cracks in the wall" in a setting where nurses may not be able to distance themselves to see the problems. And, in addition to bringing knowledge to the unit, they also take knowledge from this unit to other settings where they work, potentially impacting patient care across clinical systems.

A CASE FOR COMPLEXITY—cont'd

TNs have a unique role in this system. They provide diversity of perspective and experience, and they disseminate information and knowledge among the various clinical systems where they work. In this case, TNs delivered messages that reinforced the positive aspects of this work environment, such as the extraordinary quality of care and collaborative practice of this unit. As a result, they contributed to the improvement of patient care in this ICN as well as others. The benefits of this systems-level strategy to address the staffing needs of this unit, while controversial in some aspects, were readily apparent and multifaceted, and the nurses were pleased with the results.

Lea R. Ayers LaFave, PhD, RN; Community Health Institute/JSI

New order, novelty, chaos turning into order, and self-organization are all elements of what is termed *emergence*. New higher-level ideas, structures, and events are the result of the interaction of the lower-level components from which they emerged (Lindberg, Zimmerman, and Plsek, 2001). Martha Rogers (1970) postulated that change is the process of emergence. Wheatley (2006) grasped this concept of emergence in her description of self-organizing systems, which allow answers and change to emerge from below through relationships, information, and self-reference, rather than being imposed from the top of a hierarchy. Systems can self-organize without an imposed outside plan. The changing scientific paradigm for organizations includes these principles:

- Things do not fall apart.
- Organizations are self-organizing.
- The desired state is not equilibrium but being on the edge of chaos.
- Organizations are not things, not machines, but relationships.
- Structures emerge from these relationships rather than being imposed from the top down.
- Order is found in information rather than structure.
- Information is abundant and open, not closely managed.

Complex Adaptive Systems

Complexity science concepts coalesced into a broader view of living systems in the concept of complex adaptive systems. These are complex, nonlinear, interactive systems that adapt to changing environments. They can self-organize and are composed of many independent agents who interact at all levels. From these relationships emerge new ideas, structures, and patterns. There is surprise and unpredictability. It is at the edge of chaos that new order emerges and systems evolve while also maintaining their identities. These systems do not operate in a linear, top-down fashion but from simple rules acted upon at the local level (Lindberg, Zimmerman, and Plsek, 2001).

One important feature of complex adaptive systems is simple rules. Locally applied simple rules can result in complex outcomes. In a living system such as a flock of birds, a school of fish, or a herd of antelope, there is no identified leader. Each animal operates locally from three simple rules: (1) avoid collisions; (2) match your neighbor's speed; and (3) move toward the center of the group (Stacey, 2003). In New York City every single day, food and goods are transported in to feed millions of people. There is no food CEO, just many diverse independent agents interacting to deliver food to markets, restaurants, and kitchens. This is truly a self-organizing complex adaptive system. The simple rule is: bring in the right amount of food at the right time to the places where it is needed. The "local agents" find the information they need from the system itself, not from outside or top-down orders. There are regulations and standards to follow, but in effect they are simple rules, too.

From Science to Society and Organizations

Within a generation, complexity science evolved from the sciences of biology, physics, and mathematics and combined with early work on general systems theory to find its way into economics and organizational management. At the Sante Fe Institute in 1987, John Holland spoke about the global economy as an adaptive process. This was a turning point in relating hard science material to sociocultural organizations. Complex adaptive systems in the natural world are brains, cells, and immune systems; in the human world, complex adaptive systems are cultural and social. There are certain crucial features. There are many agents. In the brain, these are the nerve cells. In the economy, they are individuals and households. Another feature is that all the agents are in the environment, which is produced by the interactions of the agents with each other. Each agent is affected by the actions and interactions and cooperation and competition of the others. There can never be a fixed and predictable environment. Control is highly dispersed. There is no master neuron in the brain, for instance. Waldrop (1992) tells how at a Santa Fe Institute conference, Holland spoke of the economy as an example of a self-organizing system: "Ask any president trying to cope with a stubborn recession: no matter what Washington does to fiddle with interest rates and tax policy and money supply, the overall behavior of the economy is still the result of myriad economic decisions made every day by millions of individual people" (p. 145).

Field Theory

Field theory, based on even newer scientific principles, brings more understanding to how the world works and how people relate within systems. The first field theory terms were scientific terms related to electricity and magnetism. As quantum physics evolved, scientists asserted that fields underlie all matter, and they are considered regions of influence with characteristic patterns. The holistic self-organizing properties of systems at all levels depend upon morphic fields as described by Rupert Sheldrake (1995). He imagined organizations and organizational space in terms of fields, with employees as waves of energy, spreading out in regions of organization, growing in potential. Leaders are creating the fields for their organizations constantly. New leadership means creating the positive nurturing field conducive to growth and transformation.

A far more organic field is described by Mindell (1995): "Organizations are characterized not only by their overt and identifiable structure purpose and goals, but by their emotional features, such as relationships, conflicts, jealousy and envy as well as by altruistic drives, spiritual needs and interest in the meaning of life" (p. 14).

The field is the milieu for the process of relationships. Recognizing this, leaders can attend to the relationship process that will complement their structural initiatives. Senge, Kleiner, Roberts, et al., (1994) assert that one can always sense the presence or absence of leadership when entering an organization, even for the first time. A field may be one of competence and learning that, though unseen, influences behavior. They are describing Mindell's fields that, while not tangible, are felt as forces and influences.

FROM MECHANISTIC/LINEAR TO COMPLEXITY THINKING

All these concepts and theories are ways to view organizations, whether biological or social, as self-organizing systems. These are systems that may appear chaotic, but underneath they are connected by order and the capacity for self-renewal at an even higher level of complexity. Systems (organizations) are not running down but becoming better, more complex, and more connected (Wheatley, 2006).

Wheatley's work brought science and management to the same table. Her self-organizing systems approach to leadership has profound implications. No longer should we, or can we, strive for predictability and stability. It does not exist. Command and control are dissonant to those ideas. Organizations are living entities, composed of people in relationship. The old management paradigm centered on organizations as machines. Management's function was to control and manage the machine. Viewing organizations as living open systems, ever evolving toward greater complexity and order, demands different leadership. Leaders who treat people in the organization as self-organizing and self-renewing and who see the work as being accomplished through relationships are complexity leaders. Table 2–2 contrasts the features of mechanistic/linear thinking and complexity thinking about organizations.

Table 2–2	COMPARING MECHANISTIC/LINEAR AND COMPLEXITY THINKING
MECHANISTIC/LINEAR THINKING	**COMPLEXITY THINKING**
Stable and deterministic	Patterned, self-organized
Always at equilibrium	Coalescing, changing, decaying
Simple	Complex
Machine	Organism
Linear	Nonlinear
Predictable	Surprising
Controlling and controlled	Adaptable and adapting
Orderly	Patterned
Designed	Emergent
Reductionistic	Holistic
Change is troubling to the system	Change is all there is
Chaos is to be avoided	Chaos is needed for emergence
Imposed detailed direction	Self-organizing with the right simple rules

SUMMARY

Earlier in the chapter, you read some examples to consider from a complexity perspective. It should now be clearer that the fall of the Berlin Wall was the result of self-organization of many independent local agents who were drawn together by a powerful attractor: freedom. There were many voices and small local acts that contributed to the final action, but if traced back, there would not be a strong cause-and-effect relationship but a nonlinear set of conditions and circumstances. There certainly was chaos and turbulence that built and built until that final event when the wall was breached and removed very swiftly, and new order emerged from the collective endeavor.

Our second example related to the CEO who decreed a new order and structure but did not create a climate for self-organization, distributed leadership, or relationships. The CEO believed that a massive change endeavor would produce equally massive results, a very linear idea. Leaders who believe in changing the structure, whether who reports to whom or how the work is organized, are often disappointed. They do not have a complexity view. The proper understanding is that it is people in relationship who change the structure, not the other way around.

Finally, the example of an individual or small group employing small local actions to produce large systemic changes is the phenomenon of the butterfly effect. There is surprise and nonlinearity. Local agents in relationship are the ones who can truly transform a system. A most dramatic event with worldwide cascading ramifications was the Tunisian vendor who set himself on fire to protest government oppression in December of 2011. This is widely seen as the impetus for the ensuing uprising in the Middle East called the Arab spring, indeed a butterfly effect.

This chapter has laid down the foundation for science and its history, contributing to a view of organizations as living complex adaptive systems. There are terms to describe this phenomenon of living, working, and leading in the complex world of health care. Chapter 3 pulls these discrete concepts together, describing complex adaptive systems and their application to organizations.

2-1   CRITICAL THINKING EXERCISE

In an organization with which you are familiar, is the leadership thinking more linear or complex? Based on your assessment, choose two or three concepts from Table 2–2 that contrast mechanical/linear and complexity thinking, and write a short piece that describes that organization.

2-2   CRITICAL THINKING EXERCISE

Look back at this chapter's *A Case for Complexity*. Where in this case can you see evidence of emergence, self-organization, adaptability, independent agents, and distributed leadership? Describe these. As you review the concepts in this chapter, are there others that might apply to this situation?

QUESTIONS FOR SELF-REFLECTION

1. Can you recall a situation in health-care practice in which simple rules worked better than long, complicated policies and procedures? Describe that situation.
2. Have you been witness to a time in your organization when a butterfly effect launched rumors or dissention? Recall that experience.
3. Have you ever walked into a meeting or onto a patient care unit and experienced a certain feel to the field? Describe that event.

REFERENCES

Capra, F. (2002). *The hidden connections.* New York: Doubleday.

Capra, F. (1996). *The web of life.* New York: Doubleday.

Eoyang, G.H. (1997). *Coping with chaos: Seven simple tools.* Circle Pines, MN: Lagumo.

Gleick, J. (1987). *Chaos: Making a new science.* New York: Penguin.

Institute of Medicine of the National Academies. (2001). *Crossing the quality chasm.* Washington, DC: The National Academies Press.

Jantsch, E. (1980). *The self-organizing universe.* Oxford: Pergamon Press.

Lindberg, C., Zimmerman, B., & Plsek, P. (2001). *Edgeware: Complexity resources for health care leaders.* Bordentown, NJ: Plexus Institute. Retrieved April 8, 2010, from http://www.plexusinstitute.org/edgeware/archive/think/

Mindell, A. (1995). *Sitting in the fire: Large group transformation using conflict and diversity.* Portland, OR: Lao Tse Press.

Newman, M. (1994). *Health as expanding consciousness* (2nd ed.). New York: National League for Nursing Press.

Peat, D. (1990). *Einstein's moon: Bell's theorem and the curious quest for quantum reality.* Chicago: Contemporary Books.

Ray, M.A., Didominic, V.A., Dittman, P.W., et al. (1995). The edge of chaos: Caring and the bottom line. *Nursing Management, 26*(9), 48–50.

Rogers, M. (1970). *An introduction to the theoretical basis of nursing.* Philadelphia: F.A. Davis.

Senge, P.M., Kleiner, A., Roberts, C., et al. (1994). *The fifth discipline fieldbook: Strategies and tools for building a learning organization.* New York: Doubleday.

Sheldrake, R. (1995). *Seven experiments that could change the world.* New York: Riverhead Books.

Stacey, R.D. (2003). *Strategic management and organisational dynamics.* Harlow, United Kingdom: Pearson Education Ltd.

Waldrop, M.M. (1992). *Complexity: The emerging science at the edge of order and chaos.* New York: Simon and Schuster.

Watson, J. (1979/2008). *Nursing: The philosophy and science of caring* (rev. ed.). Boulder: University Press of Colorado.

Wheatley, M.J. (2006). *Leadership and the new science: Discovering order in a chaotic world.* (3rd ed.). San Francisco: Berrett-Koehler Publishers.

Wheatley, M.J. (1995). *Self-organizing systems conference.* Sundance, UT.

Wheatley, M.J., & Kellner-Rogers, M. (1996). *A simpler way.* San Francisco: Berrett-Koehler Publishers.

3

HEALTH-CARE ORGANIZATIONS AS COMPLEX ADAPTIVE SYSTEMS

Complexity leaders are ready for surprises, nonlinear interaction, feedback, and innovations through self-organization.

■ OBJECTIVES

- Apply concepts of complex adaptive systems to health-care leadership situations.
- Analyze nursing and health care within a framework of complex adaptive systems.
- Compare and contrast linear and complexity approaches to leadership.
- Discuss the dynamics of organizations with congruent or incongruent complexity/linear leadership configurations.

INTRODUCTION

This chapter takes the discrete concepts of complexity science and expands into the broader context of complex adaptive systems. Going into more depth, there are examples that relate to organizations and, specifically, to health-care organizations in order to enhance the complexity view. This understanding will help to develop your ability to use the language and to start thinking like a complexity leader. The key features of complex adaptive systems will be described with some examples to explain applicability to health-care organizations. An interesting concept to consider is the shadow system in an organization. There is also a compilation of primary complexity concepts listed as machine-versus-complexity organizational paradigms and linear-versus-complexity leadership approaches. Finally, the chapter includes the linear/complexity organizational and leadership matrix assessment tool for describing an organization and assigning the level of complexity.

COMPLEX ADAPTIVE SYSTEMS

Complex adaptive systems are nonlinear interactive systems that can learn and adapt to changing environments. They are composed of many diverse and independent agents, all in relationship; cooperating, collaborating, competing, and connecting. From the relationships emerge new behaviors and novel ideas, structures, and patterns. There is surprise and unpredictability. It is at the edge of chaos (where there is often the greatest turbulence) that new order emerges. Action takes place at the local level based on simple rules. Leadership is distributed throughout, and the system is self-organizing.

Key features of a complex adaptive system are listed and described here.

- Diverse independent agents interact and adapt to change locally.
- New behavior, ideas, patterns, and structure emerge from relationships.
- Results are often nonlinear, unpredictable, and surprising.
- Self-organization occurs with distributed leadership and simple rules

Diverse Independent Agents Interact and Adapt to Change Locally

It is not just the number of independent agents interacting locally but the nature of the interactions and connections. While the global characteristics of the system arise from the interactions, they cannot be traced back to one single agent but to relationships of more than one agent. For example, McDaniel and Driebe (2005) describe the quality of a surgical team as not based on the quality and skill of any one surgeon, nurse, or technician but on the whole team. Likewise, a patient care unit's quality and character is the sum of all the members' participation. These are examples of the whole being greater than the sum of its parts as well as the quality and interactions of each of its parts, the people involved. The patterns of relationships and connections result in the emergence of novelty and even newer patterns of relationships.

When parts of a system or group of people or department interact and produce a feature of the system not there when the parts were considered separately, that is called *emergence* (Smith and Stevens, 1999). For example, an interdisciplinary team on a mental health unit meets to plan a client's care. Each brings his or her own discipline's perspective, plus knowledge, experience, and personal reactions. In an effective team interaction, the resulting plan will bring in the diverse mental models of the individuals. It will be creative and medically sound and richer than any could produce alone. This mental health team example also exemplifies the locality of decision making. Rarely is there a one-size, top-down solution for a mental health client treatment plan.

Even within the team, it may be the newest, least experienced member who has the piece of information needed to more fully understand the client's dynamics. The mental health nurse's aide on the night shift may be the only one who sees the client engaging in a particular behavior. The nursing student with more time to spend with the client may be the one with whom the client shares suicidal thoughts. These are local, at-the-edge, situations.

New Behavior, Ideas, Patterns, and Structures Emerge From Relationships

In organizations, there is spontaneous emergence of new order and novelty where there are points of instability. Even an off-hand comment can trigger this instability, as it may have meaning to the hearers. The system then "chooses" to be disturbed, and information is circulated, amplified, and expanded to the point of more instability. The present structure, behaviors, and beliefs are then affected, leading to chaos, confusion, uncertainty, and doubt. As people interact around the situation, new order emerges with new meaning created collectively. In other words, people in relationship go through phases of reacting and acting to bring new meaning, order, and structure to their group or organization. These breakdowns or breakthroughs are usually accompanied by strong emotions. There are tension and crisis surrounding these events.

People can feel a sense of uncertainty and loss of control during the chaotic periods and, when the breakthrough occurs, there can often be a collective feeling of relief and excitement that is almost magical and can be termed team spirit. This relational, collective, "magical" aspect of moving though change takes place within a particular culture. Often, leaders attempt to replicate a positive intervention or innovation by taking it from another organization to impose on their own. This imposition often fails because the cultures are different. An idea or innovation works well when the concepts are introduced in the context of an organization's culture. Including people at all levels in distributed leadership so the culture enhances the innovation, not rebuffs it, is a powerful motivation for all involved. One justification for not imposing change from the outside or from the top is that no one, even a senior leader, is outside or at the top of the complex adaptive system. Everyone is embedded in the system and works in relationship with others. Many change efforts fail because the leaders think they are not part of the system and do not take into account the culture of that particular system.

Another relevant concept involves the contrast between designed and emergent organizations. Both exist, and both are essential, but they are complementary. The designed portion of an organization is related to the formal official aspects, such as standards, rules, policies, and procedures. The emergent portions are the informal communication networks, the relationships, and the connections that result in innovations and growth. Both are necessary in balance, the first to maintain the stability and identity of the organization and the second to facilitate new learning and growth (Capra, 2002).

A fascinating description of the informal system is the *shadow system*. Rumors, hallway conversations, and gossip are an integral part of the process. Leaders should pay attention to these emergent informal activities, connections, and informal information flow; often, the best new ideas arise there. This is a valuable way to find out what is happening, as issues cannot be addressed if they are not known (Lindberg, Zimmerman, and Plsek, 2001). Kelly (1994), in his description of living complex systems, calls the formal, more concrete, approach *clockware* and the informal relationships and connections *swarmware*. Clockware is akin to the linear procedures, routines, and functions needed to keep living systems stable, whereas swarmware refers to the more relationship-based networks and connections that produce novelty and change. Lindberg, Zimmerman, and Plsek (2001), in urging leaders to view their organizations through a complexity lens, suggest that using both clockware and swarmware is important to success.

Results Are Often Nonlinear, Unpredictable, and Surprising

Long-range strategic planning and data collection are designed to ensure flawless prediction of events and avoid uncertainty. But in the health-care world as well as in all organizations, there is uncertainty. Direct-care nurses will admit that few shifts and assignments in patient care turn out exactly as expected. Indeed, this is part of the challenge and excitement of nursing care. It is curious that these nurses often lose that perspective when in a leadership position. A complexity leader has the ability to balance tight planning while being open to new possibilities and understands that most changes cannot be predicted.

By virtue of being nonlinear, surprise and unpredictability are strong characteristics of a complex adaptive system. In traditional organizations, surprises and the unexpected are not only unwelcome but are often a source of distress. Leaders have often believed that, with sufficient planning and system design, more knowledge, and experience, surprises can be avoided; however, in complex organizations, that approach often hinders innovation and efficiency. Surprise and nonlinear results can be expected in health-care organizations as the natural order of things (McDaniel and Driebe, 2005).

Complexity leaders see opportunities for exploration in the unexpected, rather than reacting defensively and viewing it as a failure and a threat. Porter-O'Grady and Malloch (2007) say it well: "Leadership judgment is called leadership judgment because certainty is missing" (p. 172). What often happens in organizations is that the leaders assume that surprise happened because of insufficient information or the speed of obtaining needed data. So they respond to the event with requests for bigger and better computers and more data collection. If they make the assumption that the resulting information is absolute and correct and a surprise still happens, they will ask for more care and more vigilance and will spend their efforts to search for who is to blame. McDaniel and Driebe (2005) reflect on this situation: "However, if the assumption is that surprise often arises as the result of the fundamental unknowability of the world, we open the door for creative, innovative approaches without the mark of blame and failure. We change our relationship with the unexpected and resilience becomes a quality that is essential for effective management" (p. 270).

McDaniel and Driebe (2005) use concepts of complexity science to explain surprise in organizations. These are trajectories, bifurcations, self-organization, emergence, and co-evolution.

Trajectories

Trajectories are how things play out or the unfolding of events that are rarely predictable. They are influenced by many intervening events. Although the trajectory is sensitive to initial conditions, the positive and negative feedback in the system occur through relationships and unexpected behaviors. When there is a hospital merger, for example, key executives may leave, and the talent that was counted on to effect a successful merger no longer exists in the system, thus changing the trajectory of the merger and affecting its eventual outcome.

Bifurcations

Bifurcations in a chaotic system are the points where choices are made as to which branch or direction will be taken. Bifurcation is unpredictable. Whatever the choice, in one part of the system, there is a qualitative change in the whole system. For example, the unexpected closing of a mental health unit in a community hospital affects the quality of the whole community mental health system.

Self-Organization

Self-organization occurs frequently in a system without top-down direction, creating new systems and order. Local connections among people may change processes, leading to surprise. Nursing assistants in long-term care may organize care around residents' personalities and preferences. Their innovative care results in increased patient and family satisfaction, and even though this is a local action of independent agents self-organizing, the whole system is changed. Informal systems in health-care organizations frequently create effective improvement processes for patient care. These informal, self-organizing patient care innovations can be cultivated by leaders, if they stay attuned and embrace complexity leadership.

Emergence

Emergence is the process of independent agents interacting, leading to the system acquiring new properties that can be another source of surprise for health-care leaders. It is difficult to predict these emergent characteristics without assessing the individuals and their interactions and relationships. "Fixing" one person without addressing the group or system will not be helpful, and emergent surprises will continue. Medication error management is a prime example of the futility of blaming one person for the error without investigating the complexities of the entire medication distribution process.

Co-evolution

Co-evolution is the continuous mutual change that occurs as agents and systems interact. As one part changes, another adapts, and that influences further change. Hospitals preparing to apply for Magnet designation often discover that, as the chief nurse executive and the nursing department develop empowered, shared-governance capability to enhance professional practice and best practices, other departments change and grow likewise. This raises all disciplines to higher levels of performance and develops an often exciting, spirited common focus for excellence.

Surprise, which is inevitable in health-care organizations, can be the impetus for creativity. There is tension between established ways of doing things and the need to accomplish new things, and there is pressure to break away from old ways to find completely different ways to approach work. If leaders welcome surprise, they can be open to new solutions and to creating an environment for innovations to emerge from the interactions of many different people in the organization. Leaders can move from trying to keep surprise from happening to being open to asking how it can be used for creative change and improvement. Leaders who accept that they cannot control the system in all aspects will start to employ a different leadership style, one that focuses less on blame and more on the uncertainty that is inevitable in complex adaptive systems. Embracing uncertainty and surprise frees the organization to move and change and grow in exciting ways. "Surprise challenges and upsets us. Our natural desire to have the world be a predictable place and to be in control of situations as they unfold can lead to dysfunctional responses to surprise. We need to be actively engaged in surprise readiness. When surprise happens, we have to listen and ask, "What is going on here?" When we take complex adaptive systems seriously, surprise will be a natural gift to us, and with a welcoming attitude, creativity and learning will be at the forefront" (McDaniel and Driebe, 2005, p. 275).

Butterfly effects helps to explain surprise and unpredictability and can have positive or negative consequences. For instance, rumors or casual careless comments can be magnified and have destructive effects in a system. Someone trying a new treatment or procedure when all else has failed may lead to innovation and discoveries of positive new protocols. Some changes are predictable, and others cause butterfly effects. There are so many complex interdependent events occurring that create the current reality (Eoyang, 1997).

Be mindful that, in some situations, negative butterfly effects might be occurring when something entirely unexpected happens, and the leader receives a message not in keeping with the facts of the situation. There may be different interpretations of the same story and strong emotions concerning something that appears to be a neutral event (Eoyang, 1997). The following is *A Case for Complexity* that helps illustrate how the positive effects of a small local action by an independent agent leads to a large systems change.

Self-Organization Occurs With Distributed Leadership and Simple Rules

Healthy, productive, complex adaptive systems are connected to the world by their boundaries, or their edges. Outside influences, such as external information, materials, and energy, affect internal dynamics. The dynamics shift because this information, material, and energy disrupt the initial equilibrium. As the system starts to adapt to the distressed environment, differences are exaggerated, and there is turbulence. As the system is pushed far from equilibrium, with no obvious plan and without the control of an individual at the top, spontaneous

A CASE FOR COMPLEXITY

On a very active adolescent psychiatric inpatient unit, the professional staff tried several interventions to gain some order and to encourage patients to be responsible for their behavior. Acting independently, the housekeeper, who was tired of working in very disorganized, messy patient rooms, began putting stars on the doors of the cleanest, neatest room on the unit. Within a matter of days, the rooms were cleaner, and the adolescents were less disorderly and looking for ways to improve their surroundings. As an additional, beneficial, surprise, the patients took on more responsibility for their treatment, individually and in groups.

self-organization occurs. This results from an increase of interdependency and transforming feedback loops, which are pathways of communication and links that join different parts of the system. Each part responds to change and communication in other parts of the system, but no one part determines the change in the whole system.

Another component of a self-organizing system is diversity, or differentiation. The most adaptable and self-organizing systems are composed of many different agents, all coming together in communication and interaction to form the greater whole (Eoyang, 1997).

Diversity

The challenge for leaders is to take this understanding of complex concepts and translate it to the organizations of which they are a part. Wheatley and Kellner-Rogers (1996) conceptualize an organizational model with three domains: information, relationships, and self-reference. From these overlapping domains emerge the structure, patterns, and process. Based on self-organizing systems, their model moves away from control and structure toward people and relationships. Self-organizing systems "work" through relationships and the exchange of information while referring back to the original intent or purpose for existence, identity, or self-reference. Wheatley and Kellner-Rogers brought science and management to the same table, and their self-organizing systems approach to organizations has profound implications. No longer should managers strive for predictability and stability; they do not exist. Command and control are dissonant to these ideas.

System Control Parameters

Around the time that Wheatley was coming to the attention of business management, Ralph Stacey (1996) was bringing these concepts to organizational management and systems. He proposed that complex adaptive systems are driven by three control parameters: (1) the rate of information flow through the system, (2) the richness of the connectivity between and among agents in the system, and (3) the level of diversity within and between the cognitive schemas of the agents (mental models). He suggests that the system is influenced by and experiences changes in stability as adaptive nonlinear feedback networks pass through various states of change. Although this leads to some confusion, disorder, chaos, and turbulence, change remains within a contained structure that prevents the structure from falling apart into pattern-less behavior (Stacey, 1996). A model based on the systems control parameters is in Chapter 4.

Simple Rules

Simple rules encourage the environment for self-organization. A hospital's mission, vision, and values are types of simple rules that set the tone and give direction for individuals to be autonomous and creative.

Magnet organizations, for example, operate with simple rules built into structured empowerment. The Magnet system's Forces of Magnetism related to empowerment suggest that the organizational structure should be flat, flexible, and decentralized, with nurses involved in self-governance and decision making (ANCC, 2008).

Control

Once leaders view their organizations as complex adaptive systems, control becomes an issue. Humans feel the uncertainty and want to control things because their consciousness causes them to remember disasters of the past and to worry about future dire consequences (Briggs and Peat, 1999). Leaders need to adopt a different worldview of how an organization is managed because they may not be able to control their organizations from a mechanistic, linear perspective. But they can influence the direction in which the organization evolves (Lewin and Regine, 2000). Control is often confused with order if leadership is defined in terms of its control functions (Wheatley, 1995). Wheatley sums up complexity thinking by stating: "If people are machines, seeking to control us makes sense. But if we live with the same forces intrinsic to all other life, then seeking to impose control through rigid structures is suicide. If we believe that there is no order to human activity except that imposed by the leaders, that there is no self-regulation except those dictated by polices, if we believe that irresponsible leaders must have their hands into everything, controlling every decision, person, and moment, then we cannot hope for anything except what we already have—a treadmill of frantic efforts that end up destroying our individual and collective vitality" (1999, p. 25).

Linear Versus Complexity

It is important to remember that managing organizations from a complexity standpoint does not mean that there are no leadership instances or situations that require a more linear or mechanistic approach. Eoyang (1997) calls these "Newtonian actions of the leader." It is also called transactional leadership. Transactional leadership involves those day-to-day transactions around rules, policy, and procedures that keep an organization running smoothly and meeting regulations and quality standards.

Complexity leaders create the environment for self-organization (transformational leadership) while recognizing that transactional actions are also needed. Effective leaders will value and embrace both actions because the natural tension of the two facilitates innovation and change in the organization. Lewin and Regine (2000) reflect that complexity science does not replace mechanistic management; rather, it encompasses it in a larger context, using uncertainties to foster creative adaptation. It welcomes periods of chaos as not only natural but desirable. If old must go, and new is needed, chaos is often the road to follow.

Attractors

The scientific concept of attractors has valuable application to understanding self-organization and leadership. Attractors are like patterns of energy, such as the eddy formed in a rushing river that, in time, changes the course of the river. Plsek and Wilson (2001) suggest that instead of pushing for change and identifying "resistance," leaders should look for attractors in the system because these patterns of energy are the intrinsic motivators. The authors assert that attractors should match the group, rather than the leader. This requires careful attention to what those attractors may be. Attractors create the environment for self-organization as they draw people in.

As an example, Lehigh Valley Health Network implemented a complex adaptive strategy throughout its system to seek improvements in its financial status (Capuano, MacKensie, Pintar, et al., 2009) Terry Capuano, Senior Vice President Clinical Services, reports the story in *A Case for Complexity*.

A CASE FOR COMPLEXITY

IMPLEMENTING A COMPLEX ADAPTIVE STRATEGY TO PRODUCE CAPACITY DRIVEN FINANCIAL IMPROVEMENT

Situation and Actions

In early fiscal 2007, admissions at the 800-bed tertiary campus of Lehigh Valley Health Network, Lehigh Valley Hospital—Cedar Crest (LVH), were growing although we were not achieving our budget volume or financial projections. Our length of stay (LOS) was increasing, exceeding our budget target by 0.35 days. A 60-day turnaround was launched using a complex adaptive systems approach called swarmware. Swarmware projects are idea-driven, short-cycle, and limited-resource, with several being deployed at the same time. A turnaround team was quickly assembled and charged with fixing the primary driver of our financial underperformance, the increasing LOS. Goals to achieve the turnaround expectations were set:

• Reduce average LOS to at or below budget.
• Say "yes" to all patients through key points of access.

Length of Stay

While this focus area is obviously based on our goal, the strategies employed were not. Two experiments were designed. The medical department–based LOS report card gave our department chairs in medicine, surgery, and family practice access to overall, group, and individual physician LOS on a weekly basis, allowing availability and transparency of information. The variability and awareness of all physician data spurred discussion and generated improvement. A complex case management process, focusing on patients with an

A CASE FOR COMPLEXITY—cont'd

outlier long LOS, was designed. One case manager was added who would see the challenging longer-stay patients referred by the unit case manager, while the unit-based case manager continued to focus on the majority of patients to be discharged.

Getting to "Yes"

Our second goal of saying "yes" to all admissions or potential admissions allowed our access doors to remain open. The ability to accept inpatients was hampered by emergency department (ED) diversions, transfer center delays, and bed capacity constraints; thus our focus on these areas. The ED developed mechanisms to address surge capacity, including an electronic alert system to inform clinical stakeholders of the anticipation of diversion and use of outpatient areas for patients awaiting admission as space allowed.

Through our automated bed management system, we were able to immediately know when patients had been discharged and vacated their room. We experimented with moving the patient before or during discharge bed cleaning. The transfer center was re-scripted to change the message to "yes" on the first call from referrers. Needed communication and movement behind the scenes were done without inconveniencing referral centers with a delay or need for a second call.

Rounds by infection-control practitioners were initiated to review the necessity of isolation precautions on all patients. This allowed expeditious movement to cohort patients, promoted discontinuation of isolation, or led to decisions against placing a patient in isolation initially.

Results

Our rapid turnaround efforts produced the results needed to achieve our two goals. We reduced length of stay to 0.1 days below budget, meeting our 60-day goal. Saying "yes" to all patients through key access points was met by reducing transfer center denials to 0 in 19 days and monthly ED diversions from 110 hours to 20 hours in 60 days. By better managing our capacity, we created additional bed capacity, allowing us to accommodate community demand, exceed our budgeted admissions target, and stabilize our market share.

Terry Capuano, RN, MSN, MBA, FACHE, NE-C, Chief Operating Officer

For an overall conceptualization of the various complexity science concepts and their relationship to organizations and leadership, see Tables 3–1 and 3–2. Table 3–1 shows the contrasts between the older mechanistic-linear organizational paradigm and the new complexity organizational paradigm. Table 3–2 contrasts linear and complexity approaches to leadership.

| Table 3–1 | COMPARING OLD AND NEW ORGANIZATIONAL PARADIGMS |

PARADIGM	CHARACTERISTICS
Mechanistic organizational paradigm	Clockwork
	Machine
	We understand by dissection
	Knowledge is structures in pieces
	Organizations are structured as functions
	Work is structured as roles
	People are narrowly skilled
	Motivation is external
	Change is the troubling exception
	Designed
	Linear
	Controlled and controlling
	Predictable and orderly
	Leaders are above/outside the others
	The boss is an objective outside observer
	Employees are rule-following parts of the machine
	Change occurs by way of rational actions of managers
Complexity organization paradigm	Parts are understood only in terms of the whole
	Organizations are whole systems
	Work is flexible and boundary-less
	Motivation is based on connection to the whole
	Organism-like
	Nonlinear
	Surprise
	Patterned
	Adaptable and adapting
	Emergent
	Change is all there is
	There is no leader control
	Leaders are embedded in the system
	There are no observers
	It is a field out there
	We are each other's environment
	Chaos and change are the order of the day
	Changing the structure will not change the people
	The people in relationship with each other will change the structure
	Information—self-reference—relationships
	Diversity and interdependence

Table 3–2	COMPARING OLD AND NEW LEADERSHIP APPROACHES
PARADIGM	**CHARACTERISTICS**
Linear leadership actions and approach	Management by objective Individual accountability without a systems view Preference for "yes men" Lack of respect for individual employees Secrecy regarding management decisions Lack of innovation Undue attention to internal procedures and policies Plan-Organize-Control-Direct management Long-term fixed strategic planning Designed Controlled Predicted Blame Micromanaged Information not shared
Complexity leadership actions and approach	Mix cooperation with competition Control from the bottom up Grow by changing Maximize the fringes at the local level Seek persistent disequilibrium Change changes itself Create opportunities for people to form rich relationships Reduce hierarchy Free flow of information Emphasize people's self-organizing creativity Encourage differentiation Employ motivational attractors Remove barriers to self-organization Reinforce self-organizing trends Employ influence rather than control Embrace and learn from surprise Use simple rules for vision and direction Create an environment that cultivates emergence

THE LINEAR/COMPLEXITY ORGANIZATIONAL AND LEADERSHIP MATRIX

Organizations are in various stages of development in how they function, from very linear to complex. When senior leadership embraces complexity and sets the tone, the organization will be less linear and operate as a lively, creative, relationship-based, self-organizing entity. Both organizations and the people within may grow over time from linear to complexity.

Figure 3-1, the linear/complexity organizational and leadership matrix, illustrates possible configurations of organization and leadership. As the figure shows, there are four possible combinations of the linear and complexity organizational paradigm and leadership action/ approach. Quadrant 4 exemplifies the most desirable and congruent combination. Quadrant 1 is congruent, but it represents a highly linear, mechanistic structure of organization and leadership.

Quadrants 2 and 3 can be the more stressful environments because of the incongruence between the leader actions and organizational paradigm. In quadrant 2, the leader who still operates from a linear perspective can find it disorienting and confusing to work in an organization where relationships are honored and where the "messiness" of self-organization, diverse opinions, and distributed leadership is not only tolerated but encouraged. The complexity organization, however, can help the linear leader to develop and grow into a complexity leader. The quadrant 3 situation can be frustrating for complexity leaders who find themselves confined within a linear organization. But complexity

Figure 3-1 The linear-versus-complexity organization and leadership matrix.

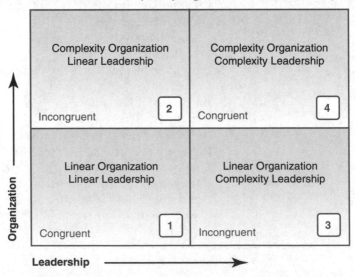

leaders have an opportunity to reach out in relationship to other like-minded colleagues to work together to transform their organization into one of complexity.

A quadrant 4 organization, the ultimate goal for complexity leaders, can be realized only if people in the organization form relationships and connections that value everyone's diverse contributions, encourage and support self-organization, encourage innovation, learn from surprise, and come together to create structure and processes that reflect their collective excellence. Of course, not all situations are pure quadrant 1 through 4, but the matrix serves as a model for reflection and assessment.

SUMMARY

The elements and characteristics of complex adaptive systems have been discussed in some detail in this chapter. The contrast of linearity and complexity paradigms for organizations and leadership was illustrated by a list of useful concepts for shifting to a complexity perspective. The linear/complexity organizational and leadership matrix is a reflective device for assessing an organization and one's place within it. Chapter 4 showcases actual contemporary applications of complexity science to nursing and health-care leadership. There is an opportunity to connect the theory in Chapters 2 and 3 to real-world health care and leadership practice.

QUESTIONS FOR SELF-REFLECTION

1. How do leaders in your organization respond to unpredicted outcomes? How do you?
2. Where do you fall on the linear/complexity organizational and leadership matrix? What feelings are evoked for you with this assessment?
3. What level of control seems to be operating in an organization with which you are familiar? How do people respond to that level of control?
4. What attractors (motivators) encourage you to do your best work?

Self-Reflection: What Have I Learned?

_____

_____

_____

_____

_____

_____

_____

_____

_____

_____

3–1   CRITICAL THINKING EXERCISE

A large health-care organization falls into quadrant 3 of the organizational leadership matrix. The organization has a history of being linear in philosophy with a senior leader (CEO) who is congruent with that hierarchical approach. It is also apparent that the CEO likes to work with his team and values its contributions. The chief nursing officer and most of the midlevel nursing directors and other discipline managers embrace many of the concepts of complexity leadership and employ these within their areas of supervision. Using concepts of complex adaptive systems, how might this group move the organization toward and finally into quadrant 4?

3–2   CRITICAL THINKING CASE FOR COMPLEXITY

I am presently working in a leadership position on a large telemetry step-down unit in a suburban hospital, and I have been thinking about our shadow system. The shadow system is the system that lies behind the scenes. It consists of hallway conversation, the grapevine, the rumor mill, and informal procedures for getting things done. Many of the staff members have been here a long time, some of them 20 years or more. The management team has two members who have also been here a long time (20 years or so), and the rest of the management team (including the educators, assistant managers, and manager) are all relatively new to the unit (1 year or less). Many changes are happening on our unit. Some of the managers are relatively new in their management roles, and two are even relatively new RNs. And, of course, there is me and my shadow! How does one deal with all these shadows? It does make for interesting dynamics.

Some other adjectives to describe the shadow system are nonlinear, innovative, creative, interesting, diverse, complex—and the system involves a larger pool of meaning, few constraints, and few rules. For example, because there are few rules and constraints, with such diverse thought, it is often the place where much creativity resides. It does not get bogged down in the bureaucratic realm like the "official system" does.

Many times the leaders of a unit view the shadow system as only negative. For example, how many times have the leaders of a unit said that their staff is resistant to change? This is an example of a military metaphor. What Ralph Stacey proposes, and I agree, is that the management of an organization should strive to embrace the shadow system instead of battling it. If management truly listens to the shadow system and embraces the shadow system, then the sky would be the limit. What diversity and innovation!

Several things intrigued me as I reflected about the shadow system. First of all, I feel that there is not just one shadow system (the staff). I feel that there are several more systems we need to look at. First is the shadow system within management. How many times have we felt as management that our peers or the people we supervise (who are also in management) are backbiting, working against us, or undermining us? It is so important that we recognize this shadow system within management. How can we supervise our staff adequately if we have undermining going on in our own ranks? The answer is that we cannot. We must be supportive of each other, recognize the shadow system within our management, and discuss issues that need to be addressed within the management so that we can effectively manage the staff. A thought—how does your management shadow system advance or impede your work?

Another key concept is that we have shadow systems within ourselves. How do we embrace our own shadows? The shadows within ourselves, the shadows within the management team, the shadows within the staff? One key principle is identification of these shadow systems, identification of the issue at hand. What aids in complexity science would assist us in embracing our shadows? One key aid is reflection. This is the art of temporarily detaching oneself from a situation in order to think clearly about it, assign interpretation and meaning to the situation, and draw out deeper knowledge.

Another aid to assist us with our shadows is the use of multiple perspectives. This involves seeing other people's perspectives and making sure the situation is safe for everyone. Participants must be open to learning how others view people and situations and must also be open to sharing honestly with others.

Uncovering and working with paradox and tension is of great help. The shadow system and the formal system in an organization are paradoxical and can be tension-filled. One must not shy away from this as if it is unnatural. Effective change has the best chance to emerge at the point of greatest tension and apparently irreconcilable differences. Do not smooth over these differences, which is what typical management often wants to do. We should focus on the differences and seek a new way forward.

A key aid is using wicked questions. Wicked questions are used to expose the assumptions we hold about an issue or situation. Articulating these assumptions provides an opportunity to see the patterns of thought and bring the differences in a group to the surface. These patterns and differences can be used to discover common ground or to find creative alternatives for stubborn problems. Wicked questions can be used by management so we can change the role of leadership from having the answers to having the questions. They can be used to open up possibilities that are not intuitively obvious, to promote ongoing inquiry, to make things permissible to discuss, to openly contrast goals and actual circumstances, to bring in new information to a problem or issue by exposing the differences. Some wicked questions that I have asked at our leadership meetings that related to this included, "How can we give direction without giving directives? How can we lead by serving? How can we maintain our authority without having control? How can we, as a large organization, be small?"

The shadow system that exists within the staff is essential to address. How does one deal with this? I truly do value the staff members and their input. I do not want them to leave. They have a wealth of experience, knowledge, and history on this unit. In a discussion with other leaders, it was suggested that in fact many of us may be staff RN haters. Wow—what a commentary and an example of our own shadows. We strive to better ourselves to get out of the staff RN role. We work to get our master's degree or to get that promotion to get off the floor. How can we be effective managers if we don't value the role of the staff RN? I worked on the floor the other day (as a staff RN) and let a staff member work my role. This was really valuable. I told the staff at our huddle meeting at the beginning of the shift what the plan was for the day. I told them to direct their concerns to Mary, the person who was going to do charge that day. I told them that I would be working the floor and might need their help (since I have not worked the floor in quite a while). In fact, I did need their help! And they were delighted to help me! They asked me how I liked working the floor, and I very honestly told them I loved it. I have altered the schedule so that I will do this about once every 2 weeks. The staff loved it.

In summary, one needs to listen to the shadow system. One needs to listen to all their shadow systems. Realize it is just a natural part of the larger system. Sometimes these shadow systems have stronger relationships than the more official system in place. Management should not try to discredit or combat the shadow systems in its organizations. Instead, we should embrace the shadows! We should use these shadows to increase the flow of information and communication, obtain varied opinions, and gain a wide range of diverse, multiple perspectives. If we embrace our shadows, I truly do believe the possibilities are limitless!

3–3   CRITICAL THINKING QUESTION   ▰▰▰

Think about your own work situation. Describe the shadow system as you see it. Is it acknowledged? How is it handled? How might it be addressed more effectively?

REFERENCES

American Nurses Credentialing Center. (2008). *Application manual: Magnet recognition program.* Silver Spring, MD: Author.

Briggs, J., & Peat, D.F. (1999). *Seven life lessons of chaos.* New York: Harper Collins.

Capra, F. (2002). *The hidden connections.* New York: Doubleday.

Capuano, T., MacKensie, R., Pintar, K., et al. (2009). Complex adaptive strategy to produce capacity-driven financial improvement. J *Healthcare Manage, 54*(5), 307-318.

Eoyang, G.H. (1997). *Coping with chaos: Seven simple tools.* Circle Pines, MN: Lagumo.

Kelly, K. (1994). *Out of control: The rise of neo-biological civilization.* Reading, MA: Addison Wesley.

Lewin, R., & Regine, B. (2000). *The soul at work.* New York: Simon & Schuster.

Lindberg, C., Zimmerman, B., & Plsek, P. (2001). *Edgeware: Complexity resources for health care leaders.* Bordentown, NJ: Plexus Institute.

McDaniel, R., & Driebe, D.J. (2005). *Uncertainty and surprise in complex systems.* Heidelberg, Germany: Springer Verlag.

Plsek, P.E., & Wilson, T. (2001). Complexity science: Complexity, leadership, and management in healthcare organizations. *BMJ, 323,* 746-749.

Porter-O'Grady, T., & Malloch, K. (2007) *Quantum leadership* (2nd ed.). Sudbury, MA: Jones & Bartlett Learning.

Smith, T.S., & Stevens, G. T. (1999). The architecture of small networks: Strong interaction and dynamic organization in small social systems. *Am Sociol Rev, 64*(3), 403-420.

Stacey, R.D. (1996). *Complexity and creativity in organizations.* San Francisco: Berrett-Koehler.

Stacey, R.D. (2003). *Strategic management and organisational dynamics.* Harlow, UK: Pearson Education.

Wheatley, M.J. (1999/2006). *Leadership and the new science: Discovering order in a chaotic world.* (3rd ed.). San Francisco: Berrett-Koehler.

Wheatley, M.J. (1995). *Self-organizing systems conference.* Sundance, UT.

Wheatley, M.J., & Kellner-Rogers, M. (1996). *A simpler way.* San Francisco: Berrett-Koehler.

4

HEALTH-CARE ORGANIZATIONAL STUDIES, THEORIES, AND MODELS BASED ON COMPLEXITY SCIENCE

Complexity leaders engage with each other to co-create an environment that honors paradox and respects all contributions.

■ OBJECTIVES

- Discuss organizational research theories and models based on complexity science.
- Apply selected theories and models to nursing and health-care leadership situations.
- Describe the role of paradox in complex leadership situations.
- Discuss the connection between effective relationships and positive patient care outcomes.

INTRODUCTION

This chapter describes several studies and models created by health-care professionals. These studies provide the evidence that the science and theory of complexity are now well incorporated into health-care professional practice across the country. All of these research endeavors and models are active, evolving projects that meet contemporary health-care leadership needs and continue to integrate complexity science into current health practice. Joyce Clifford introduced the notion of paradox in nursing administration in the early 1980s. A generation later, Tregunno and Zimmerman illustrated this from a complexity perspective. Patricia Ebright and colleagues are changing the way nurses' work is perceived, both addressing its complexity and starting the development of methods to help beginning nurses acquire the requisite skills and knowledge for complex work in their profession. Ruth Anderson, working in nursing home management, and the Dartmouth group, with its signature microsystems model, are well accomplished in applying complexity science to health care, with positive patient care outcomes. Through its requirements, the Magnet Hospital Recognition Program exemplifies the expectations of the complexity leader.

A considerable body of work is in progress by health-care professionals—nurses, physicians, and health-care management scholars—based on the science of complexity. Interest in the topic has increased as the concepts of complexity science and complex adaptive systems were discovered to have a very relevant application to health-care systems. Nurse scholars Martha Rogers, Margaret Newman, and Jean Watson were following the work of quantum physicists well before these ideas started to gain widespread attention. Holistic nurses were finding answers in science for what they once could describe only in mystical, spiritual terms. Science gave them a clearer, firmer voice in promoting their theories.

Holland (Waldrop, 1992), speaking about economics at the Sante Fe Institute; Capra (1996, 2002), bringing forth these ideas to the general interested reader; and Wheatley (1999), articulating the new science perspective, ignited the interest of health-care scholars to search for new answers. They started to investigate the value of complexity science to describe, explain, and predict health-care and patient-care outcomes. The idea that the quality of relationships within the health-care team influences the quality of health-care outcomes was beginning to take hold as a legitimate area of study.

A COMPLEX ENVIRONMENT

Ebright and her colleagues (2003) set out to investigate nurses' work environments in response to nursing shortages. They wanted to identify issues and develop strategies to help nurses maintain safety, detect patient complications, and carry out physician orders in a timely manner and to work collaboratively with other team members. Using the Human Performance Framework, in which the sharp end is the point of service and the blunt end is the resources that either facilitate or constrain the work, the research question asked was what human and environmental factors affect decision making by expert medical-surgical acute care nurses.

The cognitive factors of knowledge, mindset, and goal conflicts influence nurses. They are also affected by the complexities in the workplace: obstacles, hazards, and behaviors. To manage the complexity, nurses adapt, anticipate, accommodate, react, and cope. Observations and semi-structured interviews were used to discover (1) human and environmental issues affecting registered nurses (RNs) in work situations, (2) specific cognitive factors driving RN performance and decision making, and (3) strategies by experienced RNs to manage work successfully. Three patterns were discovered: work complexity, cognitive factors driving performance and decision making, and strategies used to manage care situations.

The team identified a key concept called *stacking*, a workload strategy for dealing with task complexities. The experienced RN is the most skilled at this behavior. As study by Ebright and her colleagues continues about stacking, they have included the concepts of *mindfulness* and *sense-making*. Their most current definition, presented at the Maine Nursing Summit on April 8, 2009 and used with permission, is: "RN stacking is a dynamic cognitive decision making process resulting in care delivery priorities, and dependent on the ability of the nurse to be mindful and engage in accurate sense-making about clinical and workflow data in the midst of unpredictable and constantly changing situations."

The challenge is to find ways to develop new graduates' skills to the point that they can become mindful and accurate in sense-making. The need for nurses who are knowledge workers, systems thinkers, and complex adaptive system managers has been identified, and the authors conclude that fundamental redesign of systems and nursing education and orientation based on understanding of the actual work is needed to support nursing work in complex systems.

STACEY MATRIX

Organizational theorist Ralph Stacey (Lindberg, Zimmerman, and Plsek, 2001) described approaches to leadership and decision making. Stacey suggested that the conditions and situations involved can help to determine the leadership actions required (Fig. 4-1).

There are times when there is clear agreement among the people involved about a course of action. Participants are very certain about the outcomes of the action and are in full agreement. More mechanistic, linear approaches, such as the plan, organize, control, and direct method, can serve well in such a circumstance. Certainty is present when there is a strong cause-and-effect linkage or in situations where positive experiences occurred in the past. At the farther end of the spectrum, chaos may dominate as all agreement and certainty dissolves. This, too, can be a time for more directive leadership to bring some outside order to a chaotic situation.

However, once a situation starts to shift from high certainty and close agreement into less certainty and agreement, it enters the zone of complexity. A complexity perspective will help leaders see that the outcome is uncertain, not controllable, so a mechanistic approach may not work. It is in those situations that leadership actions help create an environment allowing the many diverse agents in the system to connect in relationship and self-organize so that novel ideas can emerge.

There is a tendency for leaders to reverse these interventions and seek control when diversity and openness would set a better tone for creative relationships and emergent solutions. Or they will allow too

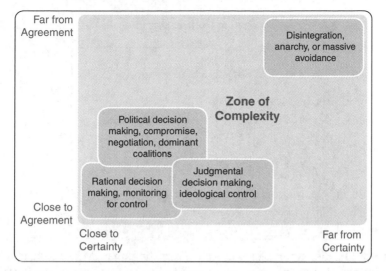

Figure 4-1 The Stacey Matrix. (Adapted from Lindberg, C., Zimmerman, B., & Plsek, P. [2001]. *Edgeware: Complexity resources for health care leaders.* Bordentown, NJ: Plexus Institute.)

much vagueness and less direction when a simple, clear policy or solution will do because the situation is certain and all agree already.

ORGANIZATIONAL DECISION-MAKING MODEL

Kinnaman and Bleich (2004) built upon the Stacey matrix with their Organizational Decision-Making Model (Fig. 4-2). This model differentiates interdisciplinary behavior in health-care organizations and was primarily aimed at the challenge of academic-service partnerships. The model assumes that not all organizational decisions are of equal concern or would necessarily require equal resources. The four concepts embedded in the diagram are toleration, coordination, cooperation, and collaboration. Each is considered for appropriate use and effectiveness based on the complexity of the initiating event and the level of agreement and certainty within the context in which the condition arises.

- *Toleration* occurs with automatic routine behaviors, where in expected circumstances people assume their roles without conscious effort, engagement, or interaction.
- *Coordination* is when two or more people provide services and work in a parallel fashion, with information being exchanged through documentation, policies, and procedures.
- *Cooperation* occurs when people work to achieve shared objectives in relationship, with the unique role and perspective of each person taken into consideration in the context of the situation.

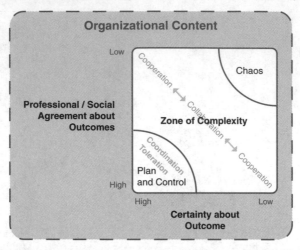

Figure 4-2 The Kinnaman-Bleich Model. (From Kinnaman, M. & Bleich, M. [2004]. Collaboration: Aligning resources to create and sustain partnerships. *J Prof Nurs, 20*[5], 310-322.)

- *Collaboration,* the highest developmental action, is an emergent, interdependent process that focuses on the complementary knowledge skills and abilities of each of the members, beyond their specific disciplines. With a focus on achieving best outcomes, there is distributed power that may even extend beyond organizational boundaries.

This model is a framework for determining appropriate behaviors and is valuable in describing group behaviors that will be effective in a complex adaptive system. In the complexity zone, collaboration can lead to relationships in which complexity leadership emerges. For instance, the need for nursing schools and health-care organizations to give students successful clinical learning experiences is an ongoing challenge. If all parties can suspend their previous assumptions about how students learn best, what has been done in the past, and who should have the authority, they can develop new and more creative student learning experiences that benefit all. New models of clinical rotations have emerged from this type of collaboration, such as dedicated teaching units and central scheduling for area hospitals and schools.

NURSING HOMES AS COMPLEX ADAPTIVE SYSTEMS

Anderson, Issel, and McDaniel (2003) suggest that nursing homes are complex adaptive systems and, furthermore, that relationships are very powerful determinants of high-quality, long-term care. Their theoretical model has its foundation in Stacey's systems control parameters, discussed in Chapter 3. In systems that are effective, managers facilitate self-organization fueled by (1) the rate of information flow throughout the system, (2) the nature of the connections among the people, and (3) diversity of cognitive schema(mental models). The management practices used can alter a system's parameters and thus relate to better patient outcomes, as shown in Figure 4-3.

Management practices observed and measured were communication openness, participation in decision making, relationship-oriented leadership, and formalization. Communication openness is the process of increasing and improving information flow among the people in an organization. The first hypothesis is that enhanced communication openness will result in a lower prevalence of resident behavior problems, restraint use, complications of mobility, and fractures.

Participation in decision making involves increasing the number of organizational connections and relationships. More participation increases the rates of information flow and the number and intensity of connections and communication among people. With more people who have diverse perspectives participating, the decisions made will lead to better outcomes; therefore, this second hypothesis proposes that greater RN participation in decision making will relate to a lower prevalence of resident behavior problems, restraint use, complications of immobility, and fractures.

Relationship-oriented leadership fosters interconnections and enhances information flow, which influences effective self-organization. This third hypothesis states that higher relationship-oriented leadership scores will relate to a lower prevalence of resident behavior problems, restraint use, complications of immobility, and fractures.

Figure 4-3 The Anderson Model. (From Anderson, R.A., Issel, L.M., & McDaniel, R.R. [2003]. Nursing homes as complex adaptive systems: Relationship between management practice and resident outcomes. *Nurs Res, 52*[1], 12-21.)

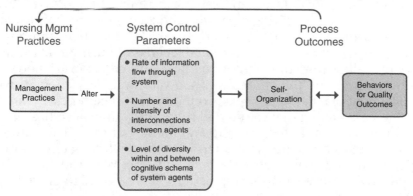

Formalization is the amount of control, rules, and regulations commonly used in nursing homes. Because of the high level of regulation inherent in the system, formalization can have the effect of suppressing self-organization, with less diversity, connection, and information flow. That leads to the fourth hypothesis, that lower formalization will relate to better patient care outcomes.

Management behaviors were observed and patient outcomes measured in 164 nursing homes. All four management practices and resident outcomes were measured and supported the influence of management practices for at least one of the four resident outcomes cited, suggesting that management practices do facilitate self-organization and can lead to better patient outcomes.

The importance of this model is its ability to serve as a framework for discussing the positive influence that best management practices can have on staff relationships and, in turn, on patient care. The nursing home culture in general is more authoritarian and confined by outside rules and regulation, and Anderson suggests that moving from the authoritarian approach to less formalization may, indeed, foster better outcomes in nursing homes.

This Nursing Management Practice Model is based on the complexity science concept that quality emerges through local interactions. Nursing management practices that facilitate new information flow, connection, and cognitive diversity are the most effective. Anderson and her colleagues continue to build upon the model with studies that investigated the relationship between management practices and outcomes such as urinary incontinence, falls, and decubuti ulcers. One contemporary work looked specifically at how managers develop relationships with and among staff that are effective in improving performance. Staff and management descriptions of management and staff relationship patterns were examined in a 6-month study in 48 nursing homes. The relationship patterns were termed local interaction strategies (LIS). From the LIS, two distinct patterns emerged: common and positive. The common pattern, which occurred more frequently, consisted of the more punitive and negative interactions such as blaming, communication breakdown, and passing the buck. The positive pattern included listening, verifying meaning, and giving respect. Some emergent characteristics of each LIS were elucidated. For the common pattern, the work environment promoted feelings of burnout, frustration, and not feeling valued. Patent care quality outcomes were poor. The positive pattern, on the other hand, showed some very effective work environment realities: teamwork, confidence, and better care planning and decision making that resulted in subsequent improved health-care outcomes. This study furthers the argument that the relationship aspects of management are essential to an optimal working environment, which then directly influences best patient care. With the discovery of the effective positive relationship pattern, it is possible to move health care toward ever-increasing positive work environments and successful patient care outcomes (Anderson et al., (2014).

Patterns of Relationship

The importance of Anderson's work is that it can be applied to all health-care settings. It illustrates how a leader's understanding about the concepts in complex adaptive systems can be used to improve the leadership and work environment through best management practices. The model brings solid, measurable aspects to an abstract body of knowledge, and it can serve as a valuable tool for nursing leaders across all levels and specialties of health care.

MICROSYSTEMS

Based in the Dartmouth-Hitchcock Medical Center, Nelson and colleagues (2002) used complexity science theory to study quality improvement in high-performing clinical units. Twenty clinical care units were studied to discover best practice ideas and the characteristics within these units that related to their high performance. The need for such a study was based on the reality that patient experiences vary widely. Staff members may work together or not; units may be in tangles or run smoothly; information may or may not be readily available and flow in a timely fashion; the units may be embedded in larger helpful or less helpful bureaucracies; the various units may be linked together or totally disjointed; and patients may find care that is high-quality, sensitive, and efficient or harmful, expensive, wasteful, and maybe lethal. This study was generated as part of the writing of the Institute of Medicine's seminal publication *Crossing the Quality Chasm* (2001).

Three assumptions about the health-care system are:

- The bigger systems are macrosystems, which comprise smaller systems, the microsystems.
- These smaller systems are the front-line producers of quality, safety, and cost outcomes.
- Macrosystems are no better than their microsystems. Each unit is embedded in a larger unit as in a fractal configuration, each unit a smaller component of the larger system.

A microsystem is defined as "A small group of people who work together on a regular basis to provide care to discrete sub-populations of patients. It has clinical and business aims, linked processes and a shared information environment, and it produces performance outcomes. Microsystems evolve over time and are often embedded in larger organizations. They are complex adaptive systems and as such they meet the needs of internal staff and maintain themselves over time as clinical units" (IOM, 2001, p. 474).

The health-care microsystem is the local milieu where patients, providers, support staff, and information processes come together to provide care. Microsystems can be tightly or loosely connected, seamless or disjointed. Some of the barriers affecting best performance and connection with the macrosystem are compartmentalization, departmentalization, and professional discipline differences that impede rather than facilitate the daily work. The microsystem with its various activities and embeddedness within other systems is influenced by regulations as well as by cultural, social, and political environments. It is a complex adaptive system evolving over time.

The research for the Nelson study included interviews, direct observations, surveys, and reviews of records. A common set of nine success characteristics were discovered: leadership, culture, macroorganizational support, patient focus, staff focus, interdependence of the care team, information and information technology, process improvement, and performance pattern. Figure 4-4 shows the Microsystem Model, and Table 4-1 reviews its success characteristics and their underlying principles. See *A Case for Complexity* on page 62.

Nelson and colleagues suggest five actions leaders can take to grow their microsystems' capacity for improvement:

- *Achieve superior microsystem results* by focusing on achieving essential outcomes, then linking to the other microsystems to meet patient, community, and business needs.
- *Use simple rules* with linked metrics to evaluate success and provide regular feedback to gauge performance.
- *Integrate information* by designing an information environment that supports the work of each microsystem for cost-effective,

Figure 4-4 The Microsystem Model. (From Nelson E.C., Batalden, P.B., Godfrey, M.M. [2007]. Quality By Design: A Clinical Microsystems Approach. San Francisco, Jossey Bass.)

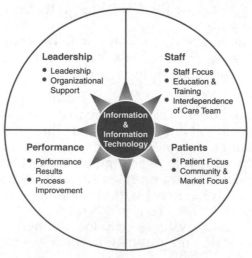

Table 4–1	SUCCESS CHARACTERISTICS OF THE MICROSYSTEM MODEL
MICROSYSTEM SUCCESS CHARACTERISTICS	**UNDERLYING PRINCIPLES**
Leadership	The leader balances setting and reaching collective goals with empowering individual autonomy and accountability.
Culture	Shared values, attitudes, and beliefs reflect the clinical mission and support a collaborative and trusting environment.
Organizational support	The leader of the organization looks for ways to connect to and facilitate the work of the microsystem and facilitates the coordination and handoffs between microsystems.
Patient focus	We are all here for the same reason: the patient.
Staff focus	There is a "human resource value chain" that links the microsystem's vision with real people on the specifics of hiring, orienting, continuously educating, retraining, and providing incentives for staff.
Interdependence of care team	A multidisciplinary care team provides care, and every staff person is respected for the vital role he or she plays in achieving the mission.
Information and information technology	Information is the connector: staff to patients, staff to staff, needs with actions to meet needs. The information environment has been designed to support the work of the clinical staff, and everyone gets the right information at the right time to do the work.
Process improvement	Studying, measuring, and improving care are essential parts of daily work.
Performance patterns	Outcomes are routinely measured, data are fed back into the microsystem, and changes are made based on the data.

high-quality care and makes for seamless handoffs between microsystems.

- *Communicate the mission* with a clear and compelling sense of organizational purpose and structure to promote and recognize high performance, linkages among the microsystems, and innovation and high-performance reinforcers.
- *Decentralize accountability* so the microsystems and the people have the decision-making capacity for their process of patient care, but provide central support for the microsystems throughout the organization (Nelson, Batalden, Huber, et al., 2002).

A CASE FOR COMPLEXITY

In an 18-month period, three interdisciplinary teams of the Elliot Health System in Manchester, New Hampshire, participated in monthly training sessions for clinical microsystems: the pain center, the endoscopy unit, and the pressure ulcer prevention team. Teams included MDs, RNs, nursing assistants, physical therapists, secretarial staff, and data analysts. One MD and one RN served as co-leaders.

A clinical microsystem is "a small group of people who work together on a regular basis to provide care to discrete subpopulations of patients." The clinical microsystems approach works on two levels. First, in order to level the playing field among the disciplines, it provides teams a structure for how to work together, such as:

- A specific format for meetings
- A proscribed improvement process that begins with assessment of the purpose, patients, professionals, processes, and patterns of the microsystems
- Templates for stating measurable global and specific aims

Second, it teaches teams improvement skills to assess and change their clinical practice, e.g., value stream mapping, fishbones, flow charts, action plans. These teams are *not* problem-focused committees. They are collaborative practice teams that meet weekly to evaluate, reflect on, and improve their practice as a unit.

This case study concerns the pain center, which redesigned its interdisciplinary pain management program (IPMP) for accreditation purposes. The center lacked outcomes for program effectiveness because it had not defined its inputs. It lacked a standard for measuring patient status before admission. The IPMP also lacked a clear structure to which changes in patient status could be attributed. The first aim was to identify evidence-based criteria for admitting patients to the program and a standardized process for admission from

A CASE FOR COMPLEXITY—cont'd

time of initial referral to team review of new patients' appropriateness for the program. The pain center developed the following:

1. Increase to 90% the number of new referrals contacted to schedule an appointment within 24–48 hours of receipt of referral; to be accomplished by June 1, 2009.
2. Increase to 90% the number of scheduled appointments within 10 business days of initial patient contact; to be accomplished by June 1, 2009.
3. Design a clear process, with criteria, for admitting 100% of appropriate patients to the IPMP; to be accomplished by July 1, 2009.

The clinical microsystems training has been successful. The team had been trying to redesign the IPMP for 2 years before the training; with training, the team accomplished it in 9 months. The team began using the new process and criteria to admit patients. This involved changing processes from the front office and through the initial visit as well as developing the structure and processes of a new clinical review team. Team members meet weekly to review charts, spending 3 minutes per chart to make admission decisions.

The team will meet as long as the IPMP exists. Its new aim is to design the process for managing patient progress through the IPMP and to identify discharge criteria. This will involve developing communication systems among clinicians of different disciplines who see patients at different sites. One team member said, "Our skills and strengths as a team have grown tremendously along the journey."

Kathleen M. Thies, PhD, RN; Gerard Hevern, MD; Jill St. Jean, RN

The Paradox of Managerial Control and Professional Autonomy

Two nurse leaders a generation apart recognized and wrote about paradox in nursing leadership, one of the more difficult concepts to grasp or appreciate while in the leadership role. Clifford and Tregunno articulate the phenomenon well.

While vice president for nursing at Beth Israel Hospital in Boston, Joyce Clifford (1981) introduced the paradox of professional-bureaucratic conflict and accountability. Clifford described the cliché of wearing two hats as the actual dilemma nurse administrators face daily: manager accountability and professional accountability. She believed that nurse leaders could honor both by maintaining identity as a professional nurse, monitoring and evaluating practice from a professional peer-group orientation, responding to patient needs, and providing opportunities for nurses to practice professionally (not just holding them to accomplishing tasks).

Clifford saw implementation of primary nursing as the way to professionalize nursing, distribute leadership, and still fulfill the classic management responsibilities. She envisioned the positive results to be mutual accountability, a sense of worth, and an environment of trust among professionals. It is instructive to see how Clifford's thinking and approach to leadership were indicative of promoting self-organization and an understanding of how her organization and nursing department were complex, adaptive systems. Clifford used complexity leadership to implement professional nursing.

Paradox in Nurse Manager Accountability

Paradox is part of a complex adaptive system by the very nature of the system. If novelty and endless variation emerge from turbulence, the paradox of two conditions is present at the same time; for example, stability and instability. With paradox, the two conditions are true, rather than contradictions or opposites. Tregunno and Zimmerman (2008) identified three paradoxes of accountability that face nurse managers. They propose that new approaches to evaluation of nurse manager accountability are needed in terms of complexity science. Nursing managers face three areas of tension (paradox) in their roles: (1) efficiency and effectiveness, (2) task and relationship, (3) stability and change.

Efficiency and Effectiveness

Nurse managers work daily with the relationships between resource inputs and clinical outputs. The pressure to do more with less is real. Nurses are accountable for manipulating staffing levels, skill mix, and patient care processes for efficiency while at the same time delivering effective evidenced-based nursing care and complying with the various professional standards, regulations, and scope of nursing practice.

Task and Relationship

Nurse managers live with the tension of attending to and being accountable for both the tasks (knowledge and competencies) and the relational aspects of nursing care and leadership. While in the health-care setting these may be viewed as two separate accountabilities, both are needed in balance to truly accomplish the management role.

Stability and Change

This is the paradox that requires the nurse manager to innovate and adapt and yet keep things on track and predictable. Change and continuity are complementary. The energy to drive change must be contained within safe guidelines for practice.

The challenge generated with these paradoxes of accountability is how to evaluate that these accountabilities are being met. Tregunno and Zimmerman propose that two different types of evaluation are needed that are tailored to the specific side of each paradox. *Summative evaluations* are rational, linear, and goal-driven, with a linear relationship between input process and output, and are based on careful protocols and data collection. Summative evaluations are effective for the efficiency, task, and stability side of the manager accountability paradox. Summative evaluations require clarity, which does not take into account emergence, surprise, and the ability to respond to unanticipated contexts. The techniques are traditional quantitative methods of judging success of outcomes based on concrete predetermined goals and compliance with prescribed and approved procedures.

For the other side of these paradoxes, (effectiveness, relationship, and change), a developmental evaluation framework may capture the accountability better. *Developmental evaluation* fits the complexity paradigm because there is a focus on short-term, desired outcomes as well as longer-term opportunities that may emerge. There is attention to the patterns that arise, and new unanticipated outcomes are welcomed. Connection and relationship are important as people learn to be open and accept that they do not have complete control of the outcomes. The developmental approach to evaluation takes into account innovation, unanticipated events, openness to emergence, and learning from feedback that will inform future actions. Table 4–2 contrasts summative and developmental evaluations with examples.

Table 4–2 · SUMMATIVE VERSUS DEVELOPMENTAL EVALUATION

SUMMATIVE EVALUATION (EFFICIENCY, TASK, AND STABILITY)	DEVELOPMENTAL EVALUATION (EFFECTIVENESS, RELATIONSHIP, AND CHANGE)
Linear	Complex
Quantitative	Qualitative
Measurable	Open to interpretation
Classic quality improvement methods	Emergent relationship-based approaches
Benchmarking	Dialogue/scenarios
Data-driven research studies based on standards and regulations	Open discussion about possibilities, looking for positive patterns with appreciative inquiry

THE MAGNET MODEL

Although not originally developed as a complexity model, the ANCC Magnet Recognition Program Model can be described in complexity science terms. When hospitals and their nursing departments arrive at the end of their Magnet journey, if successful (or even if not fully successful), they will see that they have accomplished their goal with actions and activities that are complexity-based. With Magnet status, they have become organizations that fit the organization and leadership matrix (described in Chapter 3) for quadrant 4: congruent complexity leadership in a complexity organization.

The Magnet Model has empirical outcomes in its center. The other four components—transformational leadership; structured empowerment; exemplary professional practice; and new knowledge, innovations, and improvement—are all achieved with activities based on complexity science characteristics.

The Magnet Chief Nursing Officer (CNO) is a transformational leader who is visible and accessible and who uses relationships to advocate for nurses throughout the organization at all levels and in all disciplines. The CNO develops structures, processes, and expectations for staff nurses' input and involvement. Nurses at all levels of the organization should perceive that their voices are heard, input valued, and practice supported. The free flow of information and relationship-based communication are Magnet and complexity leadership qualities.

The structured empowerment component of the model exemplifies the complexity paradigm. It calls for a Magnet environment that is generally flat, flexible, and decentralized. Nurses are supported in decision making within a self-governance structure.

The exemplary professional practice component is driven by interdisciplinary collaboration. Professional practice ensures that nurses have autonomy and control of their own practice, staffing, and schedules.

The new knowledge, innovation, and improvements component recognizes that organizations cannot stand still but should be ever-changing to higher levels of practice. "Establishing new ways of achieving high quality, effective and efficient care is the outcome of transformational leadership, empowered structures and process and exemplary professional practice in nursing" (ANCC, 2008, p. 50). Performance measures, data collection, and analysis that lead to ever increasing successful outcomes are expected of Magnet Organizations. One vehicle for creating this culture of inquiry is the partnership formed in 2011 between the Journal of Nursing Administration (JONA) and the Magnet Recognition Program. Knowledge building for nurses at all levels is facilitated, thus creating the impetus for ever improving nursing care outcomes.

Magnet organizations are environments created for self-organization, distributed leadership, free flow of information, and connection across all levels, as well as autonomous action at the local point of service level. A CNO contemplating starting the Magnet journey may be served well by striving to fulfill the role of complexity leader. Performance measures, data collection, and analysis that lead to ever-increasing successful outcomes are expected of magnet organizations. One vehicle for creating the culture of inquiry is the partnership formed in 2011 between the *Journal of Nursing Administration* (JONA) and the Magnet Recognition Program. Knowledge building for nurses at all levels is facilitated, thus creating the impetus for ever-improving nursing care outcomes.

SUMMARY

This concludes Unit One, in which the Complexity Leadership Model was introduced and described as the framework for this text. The first component of the model, knowledge of complex adaptive systems, was presented as the theoretical foundation needed to learn about organizations and develop a complexity perspective. Chapter 2 contained some historical background and discrete concepts of complexity science. Chapter 3 applied these to organizations, and Chapter 4 describes contemporary applications of the complexity foundation.

Unit Two focuses on leadership, the second major component of the Complexity Leadership Model. Chapter 5 relates the history of leadership and leadership theory. Chapter 6 moves to contemporary leadership models that contributed the complexity perspective of leadership. Chapters 6 and 7 are dedicated to knowledge and interventions that support the complexity leader.

QUESTIONS FOR SELF-REFLECTION

1. Do you know how to recognize a situation that does not require extensive group discussion?
2. When assembling a work group or task force, do you choose people who think and act like you, or do you seek diversity? Which is more comfortable?
3. Do you tend to become very directive when the answer to a problem is unclear or there is disagreement?
4. Identify one paradox in your work. Describe this paradox and how you accept and work with it.

Self-Reflection: What Have I Learned?

_____

_____

_____

_____

_____

_____

_____

4–1 CRITICAL THINKING EXERCISE ■■■■■■■■

An assumption in complexity leadership thinking is that the quality of relationships influences the quality of patient care outcomes. This was hard to justify until current nursing and health-care professionals conducted research. Choose a model presented in this chapter, and write an exemplar that applies the model's practices of leadership to a health-care organizational leadership situation, and demonstrate how patient care may be improved.

4–2 CRITICAL THINKING CASE FOR COMPLEXITY ■■■■■■■■

At a community hospital, an orthopedic surgeon requested a disposable blood pressure cuff for each total joint patient upon admission, citing the risk of contracting a nosocomial infection. Evidence for infections caused by transmission from contaminated equipment was minimal, although the literature regarding the rise of infections was abundant. Key players were identified and invited to a brainstorming session. Attendees included representation from infection control, risk management, environmental services, materials management, and nursing. The surgeon chose not to attend but was kept informed of the results of the group meetings.

At the initial meeting, the surgeon's request was presented to the group. Although everyone agreed to the proposed concept, no one agreed that disposable blood pressure cuffs were the best solution. What would meet the needs of the surgeon and, most important, the safety of the patients? Some ideas presented included addressing all shared medical equipment, enforcing policies and procedures regarding cleaning of equipment, using reusable cuffs, or purchasing disposable cuffs. After much debate, which included the cost and environmental impact of disposable blood pressure cuffs, the consensus was to test a small population of patients with a reusable cuff. All surgical patients were given an appropriately sized reusable cuff marked with the departments' initials. This cuff followed the patient through the perioperative course. When not in use, it was attached to the patient's bedrail for easy access. Once the patient was discharged, the cuff was placed in a container and picked up by a staff member from the central sterile department. The cuffs were cleaned with a germicidal solution and returned to the appropriate department.

The results were positive and, after 6 months, the remaining nursing units also implemented this process. Each department purchased its own cuffs and put the department name on them. If a patient was transferred to another unit, the cuff would follow the patient. Once the patient was discharged, the cuffs were manually cleaned and returned to their original location.

Patients expressed their satisfaction with receiving their own blood pressure cuff. The initiating surgeon was pleased that patients' needs were met. The staff, too, was satisfied. They were happy that each patient had the correct size cuff readily available when needed. The overall process improvement initiative was successful.

Denise Timberlake, RN, BSN, CNOR, Perioperative Nurse Manager

4–3 CRITICAL THINKING QUESTION

Refer to the Stacey Matrix. Describe how the case above exemplifies the theory behind the matrix as well as other complexity concepts.

REFERENCES

American Nurses Credentialing Center. (2008). *Application manual: Magnet recognition program.* Silver Spring, MD: Author.

Anderson, R.A., Issel, L.M., & McDaniel, R.R. (2003). Nursing homes as complex adaptive systems: Relationship between management practice and resident outcomes. *Nurs Res, 52*(1), 12-21.

Anderson, R.A., Toles, M.P., Corazzini, K., et al. (2014). Local interaction strategies and capacity for better care in nursing homes: A multiple case study. *BMC Health Serv Res, 14,* 244.

Capra, F. (2002).*The hidden connections.* New York: Doubleday.

Capra, F. (1996). *The web of life.* New York: Doubleday.

Clifford, J.C. (1981). Managerial control versus professional autonomy: A paradox. *J Nurs Adm, 11*(9), 19-21.

Ebright, P., Patterson, E., Chalko, B, et al. (2003). Understanding the complexity of registered nurse work in acute care settings. *J Nurs Adm, 33*(22), 630-638.

Hill, K. (2002). From the editor: The art of communicating outcomes. *J Nurs Adm, 42*(10), 50.

Institute of Medicine of the National Academies. (2001). *Crossing the quality chasm.* Washington, DC: The National Academies Press.

Kinnaman, M. & Bleich, M. (2004). Collaboration: Aligning resources to create and sustain partnerships. *J Prof Nurs, 20*(5), 310-322.

Lindberg, C., Zimmerman, B., & Plsek, P. (2001). *Edgeware: Complexity resources for health care leaders*. Bordentown, NJ: Plexus Institute. Retrieved April 8, 2010, from http://www.plexusinstitute.org/edgeware/archive/think/

Nelson E.C., Batalden, P.B., Huber, T.P., et al. (2002). Microsystems in health care: Part 1. Learning from high-performing front-line clinical units. *Joint Commission J Quality Improvement, 28*(9), 472-497.

Tregunno, D., & Zimmerman, B. (2008). The Möbius band: Paradoxes of accountability for nurse managers. In C. Lindberg, S. Nash, & C. Lindberg (eds.). *On the edge: Nursing in the age of complexity*. Bordentown, NJ: Plexus Press, pp. 159-184.

Waldrop, M.M. (1992). *Complexity: The emerging science at the edge of order and chaos*. New York: Simon and Schuster.

Wheatley, M.J. (1999/2006). *Leadership and the new science: Discovering order in a chaotic world* (3rd ed.). San Francisco: Berrett-Koehler.

Zimmerman, B. & Ng, S. (2008). Beyond the bedside: nursing as policy making. In C. Lindberg, S. Nash, & C. Lindberg (eds.). *On the edge: Nursing in the age of complexity*. Bordentown, NJ: Plexus Press, pp. 125-158.

Complexity Leadership Models, Styles, and Behaviors

5

HISTORICAL TRANSITION FROM CLASSIC TO COMPLEXITY LEADERSHIP

*The complexity leader knows that attempting to act on others from the
top or from outside the system yields very little.*

■ OBJECTIVES

- Describe the development of leadership theory from scientific-mechanistic to whole systems and complexity.
- Analyze the role and position of leaders in organizations within the historical context of leadership theory.
- Apply selected leadership theories to contemporary leadership in health care.
- Assess the effectiveness of restructure and quality improvement efforts in health care related to the leadership approaches of the 1990s and early 2000s.

INTRODUCTION

This chapter describes the evolution of management theory in relation to complexity leadership. The key theories of management from the first industrial age, scientific management, to leadership informed by complexity science concepts are discussed. These are: human relations, behavioral, trait, style, systems, situational, and transformational. The role and placement of the leader changes over the century from being outside and above the organization, not touched or affected, to a wholly immersed, fully engaged leader in relationship with all people at all levels. From a leadership perspective, this changes everything in significant ways and facilitates complexity thinking. From the perspective of the Complexity Leadership Model, leadership style, personal being and awareness, and action are influenced by a complexity view. Figure 5-1 is a timeline of this history.

SCIENTIFIC MANAGEMENT

Scientific management was the natural outflow of the mechanistic and reductionistic approach of the scientific revolution applied to the workers in factories at the start of the Industrial Revolution. Frederick Taylor and Henri Fayol were engineers in the United States and England who were concerned with efficient performance. They considered the manager to be the objective observer of the mechanism, the organization. Taylor focused on standards, skills, work assignments, laws, rules, and principles. Fayol believed that managers took distinct actions to forecast, plan, organize, coordinate, and control by setting rules for others to follow. The plan, organize, control, and direct (POCD) paradigm has been a theme of management theory throughout the century and continues in some contemporary literature.

Taylor and Fayol believed that the scientific method could be applied to human actions and that managers choose the rules driving the organizational members. This was based on Kant's concept of human beings as autonomous and possessing rational causality, that they can choose their goals and the actions to achieve them. But Taylor and Fayol's scientific management theories considered that rational causality applied only to the managers, who were autonomous, and not to the workers whom they led. The managers made the choices and designed the rules. The workers were considered just rule-following parts of the organization (Stacey, 2003).

Figure 5-1 Evolution of complexity thinking.

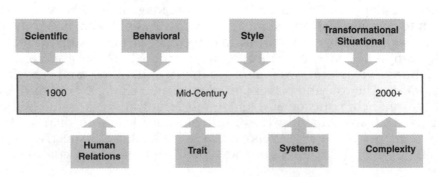

Century Timeline of Organizational Leadership

HUMAN RELATIONS/BEHAVIORAL MANAGEMENT

In what can be described as an ethical reaction to scientific management, the human relations school of management was initiated by Elton Mayo and Mary Follet, among others. They developed the ideas of humanistic and participatory management. It was Mayo's work at the Hawthorne factory from which the term *Hawthorne effect* emerged. Mayo discovered that productivity increased by just the action of paying more attention to employees. Employee motivation was studied as part of the human relations movement. With more freedom and attention to motivation, management theory moved closer to Kant's rational causality, people as autonomous. McGregor and Herzberg applied motivational theory to their behavioral models (Marquis and Huston, 2000; Stacey, 2003; Swanberg and Swanberg, 2002).

Herzberg's Hygiene and Motivation

Herzberg's two motivational factors are hygiene and motivation. Examples of hygiene factors are salary, job security, and working conditions. Examples of motivational factors are achievement, recognition, work responsibility, and advancement (Swanberg and Swanberg, 2000).

McGregor's Theory X and Theory Y

Theory X and Y was McGregor's signature motivational model. Based on Maslow's motivational model, he postulated that employees are motivated and influenced by leaders who hold one of the following assumptions:

Theory Y:

- Management is responsible and must direct, motivate, control, and modify.
- People are passive, indolent, and lack ambition, and they want to be led.
- People are self-centered and resistant to change.

McGregor's antidote to these Theory Y assumptions was *Theory X*. Managers can change their approach based on these precepts:

- Management is still responsible for the organization accomplishing the ends, the outcomes.
- People are not naturally passive or resistant but have been made that way by management.
- Management can bring out, motivate, and develop a sense of responsibility and can arrange conditions to bring out the best in people (Swanberg and Swanberg, 2000).

The one common feature of human relations/motivational theories is that they are based on the premise that managers can manipulate factors and circumstances to motivate the behavior of employees. At that time in management theory and practice, there was the prevailing notion that leaders are outside and acting on the system and the people inside.

TRAIT THEORY

The first trait theory was that of the Great Man. The basis for this thinking was that great leaders are born with leadership traits inherent in their nature. Many of the traits used to illustrate great leaders were extrapolated from observing those who were considered successful leaders. Gardner (1995) studied eleven leaders who were as diverse as Eleanor Roosevelt, Alfred Sloan, and Gandhi, and concluded that there are four factors essential for effective leadership:

- A tie to the community or audience
- A rhythm of life that includes both immersion and isolation
- A relationship between the stories leaders tell and the traits they embody
- Arrival at power through choice of the people rather than brute force

These traits have the quality of the complexity leader: relationship-based and self-reflective.

LEADERSHIP STYLES

Two classic and similar leadership style theories were those of Likert and Lewin. Likert labeled his four approaches exploitive-authoritarian, beneficent-authoritarian, casual-democratic, and participative-democratic. Lewin named his leadership styles authoritarian, democratic, and laissez-faire. (Marquis and Huston, 2000; Stacey, 2003; Swanberg and Swanberg, 2002). Both illustrate the progression of styles from highly directive to less directive and propose that, in general, a democratic-participatory style is the most effective.

This is the beginning of management theory that values workers' participation. Leaders in human relations management move closer to the people they lead. But there is the theme of the leader choosing the style and action from a position of authority and still somewhat removed from relationships with others.

SYSTEMS THINKING AND SYSTEMS THEORIES

The scientific revolution set the stage for the Industrial Revolution as more and more machines and mechanisms were invented. The

Newtonian concept of the machine-like universe was counterbalanced in the 19th century by philosophers Hume and Kant. Hume did not see knowledge as just objective and rational, but relative and subject to personal interpretation. Hume was addressing the question of human knowing. Kant was interested in human freedom and choice. He questioned whether people can have freedom and choice if they are just part of a machine-like deterministic world.

Hume and Kant's philosophy is important to understanding the history of management theory and how it evolved from mechanistic to complex. Of particular importance is how the role of the leader was first viewed as outside of and manipulating the system and then viewed as immersed within and part of the system. Kant tackled both the nature of human knowing and human freedom and choice. Stacey (2003) considers Kant to be the originator of systems thinking, which, in turn, is the forerunner of complexity science theory.

Kant conceptualized individuals as autonomous and operating in a living natural system, and he was the first to refer to organizations as self-organizing systems. His view, which was taken further by von Bertalanffy and others, explained self-organization as a way to maintain or unfold an already predetermined system whole. This view of self-organization was very important to the scientific world and to those who applied it to organizations as well. But this explanation did not take novelty into account; thus, novelty was formative rather than transformative. A formative system cannot account for surprise, unpredictability, and new emerging order from relationships (Stacey, 2003).

Three schools of systems thinking were being developed at about the same time, the 1940s to the1960s. These were general systems theory, cybernetics, and systems dynamics. General systems theory, von Bertalanffy's major work, was founded on the concepts of home-ostasis. The system was always moving to a state of order and stability through the activity of importing and exporting from other systems but essentially staying the same.

Cybernetics describes systems as adapting to their environment through self-regulation, a form of negative feedback. One everyday example of negative feedback is that of the house thermostat. The difference between the actual temperature in a room and the set temperature triggers the furnace to turn on to bring the heat up to the set temperature. The system is trying to maintain itself at a constant.

Systems dynamics was based on mathematical models to see how a system changes over time. A system may influence itself to sustain or even to be self-destructive. Engineers and computer scientists embraced these ideas as well as some management theorists. In many ways, these mid-20th century scientists were so enthusiastic about math and computer modeling that they moved away from Kant's thesis that individuals were autonomous beings and that it is human action that can be understood in terms of systems (Stacey, 2003).

Two management theories based on systems thinking that treated people as autonomous beings in charge of their actions were strategic choice theory and the learning organization. To a great extent, in these too, while moving closer to embracing the idea that people in relationships are important, the leader is still considered to be influencing the system from the outside. This is especially true of strategic choice theory.

Strategic Choice Theory

Strategic choice theory was derived from cybernetics systems thinking and the idea that one can control the way human beings perform a given pattern. The theory is based on negative feedback, where the outcomes of a previous action are compared with some desired outcome. The discrepancy is addressed in order to close the gap between the actual and the set goal. Quality improvement is a prime activity that exemplifies negative feedback with setting standards, measuring, and redoubling efforts to meet goals. With strategic choice, the strategy of an organization and its general direction are chosen by the most powerful individuals in that organization. They design the system and assign the roles, objectives, and activities needed to achieve the selected strategies. One important assumption in strategic choice theory is that it is possible for the powerful people to stand outside the organization as objective observers and control the actions of others.

Some of the tools used with strategic choice are very familiar in contemporary health-care organizations. These include financial performance measures; cost-benefit analysis; product life cycle; and strengths, weaknesses, opportunities, and threats (SWOT). Another familiar management method based on strategic choice theory is management by objectives (MBO). Strategic choice does not take into consideration culture, political messages, power, motivation, and leadership skills. It has been effective in improving efficiency and quality in health care. Strategic choice still assumes that leaders are objective observers and can determine and predict outcomes and prevent surprise and disorder. Paradox is not taken into account as it is expected that a system can eliminate or resolve all tensions, conflicts, and dilemmas (Stacey, 2003).

Learning Organization Theory

Chris Argyris (1991) and Peter Senge (1990) popularized learning organization theory. Important insights were gained by leaders who studied and applied their work. Argyris's double-loop learning was a major revelation that helped leaders implement real growth and change. Single-loop learning is similar to negative feedback, whether that is the living room thermostat or classic quality management techniques of setting standards, measuring, and then ramping up efforts to meet the standard if it falls short of the goal. Single-loop learning does not take into account the human factors, emotions, and relationships that might influence outcomes.

Argyris describes how difficult it is for even a group of very intelligent people to become a learning organization. Double-loop learning can help. Powerful, intelligent people make two mistakes: They define learning as just problem-solving, and they go about identifying and correcting errors that are caused by their external environment. But with double-loop learning, leaders and teams look within, to reflect upon what they, through their own behavior, may have inadvertently contributed to the problem. They then work together to change their behavior as well.

Single-loop learning is an example of a cybernetics system, negative-feedback mechanism. Double-loop learning is akin to positive feedback. In double-loop learning, the thermostat would be able to ask, "Why am I set at 68 degrees?" (Argyris, 1991). People have the capability to ask if they choose. Professionals have trouble reflecting on what part they may have played in a situation. They are so used to succeeding and meeting their goals that failure seldom happens, and they are not comfortable learning from failure. When things go wrong, they tend to get defensive, blame others, close off, and resist learning from the experience. In the financial crisis of 2008, the people in Wall Street financial firms were so engrossed in their success that they hardly questioned the outcomes or reflected on the part they may have played when things went wrong.

Double-loop learning requires what Argyris calls *productive reasoning*. When leaders resist reflection, they can develop brittleness. There is a disconnect between their espoused values and theories of action (how to think and what the rules for action are) and how they actually act. Defensive routines are used to ward off consideration of the part they may have played. Much of the dysfunction in an organization is caused by this discrepancy gap between espoused theory of action (what they say they believe is the right way to act) and the actual actions (Argyris, 1991). When leaders are personally self-reflective and come together as a group, in relationship, for self-reflection, double-loop learning can occur.

Senge's System Thinking

Senge (1990) promoted organizational learning through systems thinking. Argyris's action-oriented interventions to promote organizational learning dovetailed with Senge's promotion of organizational learning through systems thinking. Five practices or disciplines that contribute are:

- Systems thinking
- Personal mastery

- Mental models
- Building shared vision
- Team learning

Systems thinking entails viewing the organization from a systems perspective rather than from individual roles or functions. Personal mastery is important for a learning organization because it requires each individual to commit to striving for a high level of proficiency and lifelong learning. Built on Stacey's systems parameters (rate and flow of information, connections and communication, and diversity of mental models), the learning organization will understand and take into consideration individual and shared mental models. Building a shared vision is accomplished through people working together, being inspired to develop a strong shared vision of the future. Finally, team learning is based on all members opening to authentic dialogue and being willing to engage in double-loop learning (Senge, 1990; Stacey, 2003).

Senge acknowledged that these disciplines are best practiced within a relationship context, and they encompass both individual and group development. Practicing all Senge's disciplines can facilitate the learning organization. Senge asks leaders to consider whether they have a learning disability that keeps them from becoming true learning organizations. These disabilities are:

- *I am my position.* Over-identification with one's department or discipline closes off new learning such as Cross training, multidisciplinary teams, and interdepartmental collaboration.
- *The enemy is out there.* External threats from third-party payers and regulatory agencies have often been blamed in health care for change efforts that were not always thought out, with little introspection as to what internally could prompt improvements.
- *The illusion of taking charge.* An aggressive response to a situation, "taking charge" may be considered proactive, but it is really reactive. It is still reacting to the situation, whereas true proactive behavior involves looking within to how one contributed to the situation.
- *Fixation on events.* People can become focused on short-term events, therefore going for short-term solutions rather than seeing the longer-term patterns of change in the system.
- *The boiled frog.* The parable of the boiled frog is that a frog dropped into hot water will quickly jump out. But a frog placed in warm water will fail to notice the water heating up until it is too late to jump out. People tend to ignore trends and long-term patterns as they get swept up in a frenetic pace to compete and stay ahead. Seeing the greatest threats requires

slowing down to detect the subtle changes, not just reacting to the dramatic ones.

- *The illusion of learning from experience.* Many actions taken in an organization are on such a long-time horizon that it may not be possible to know what the consequences of these actions will be. This dilemma, once recognized, may free a group to realize that all the answers cannot be assured and that intuition, risk taking, or trying new things in different ways may yield more creative outcomes in the long run.
- *The myth of the management team.* Senge believes that management teams do not work much of the time. Members are so involved in protecting themselves from threat that consensus is watered down and all keep themselves from learning. This idea needs to be challenged as it is based on old management paradigms of control and turf rather than individuals committed to personal mastery, dialogue, and appreciating diverse mental models.

Senge and Argyris bring the leader more and more into the heart of the organization. When leaders take part in relationships, reflect upon their leadership practice, and take responsibility rather than observing and directing from outside or the top of the hierarchy, their practice is complexity-based.

TRANSFORMATIONAL LEADERSHIP

Transformational leadership has gained widespread recognition for its value in helping leaders became more than maintainers of a rigid organization, but change makers. Burns's (1978) work about the transforming leader was the foundation for transformational leadership models. He describes the transforming leader as one with the ability to create visions and employ charismatic behaviors. Burns described transforming leaders as purposeful leaders who seek to understand the motivation and needs of their followers. Transformational leadership generates collective purpose and can be judged effective if actual social change results. When one or more persons engage others in such a way that leaders and followers raise one another to higher levels of motivation and morality, true transformational leadership is present.

Personal transformational leadership traits focus much more on the ability to influence and implement second-order change. First-order change is change within an established system, whereas second-order change results in a change of the system itself, e.g., transformation (Watzlawick, Weakland, and Fisch, 1974). A complexity view helps leaders see the whole system and facilitate second-order change.

Dunham-Taylor (1995) discovered that effective nurse administrators had characteristics and traits of transformational leaders. They strive for higher quality, both organizationally and personally. They are comfortable with change. Their leadership is dynamic, visionary, and value-driven, and they can be very serious about their work. They possess humor, integrity, humility, and charisma. They have the capacity to be intuitive in their decision-making, are aware of their own humanity, and coach others rather than direct.

Marriner-Tomey (1993) described the actions of transformational leaders. They are able to cultivate relationships, build coalitions across lines and with people in different departments and disciplines, and use excellent communication skills. By empowering others and being trustworthy and purposeful, they engender a high level of motivation in others. Taking risks that reflect their own self-identified values, they are self-reflective, always seeking to understand their own contribution to a relationship or situation. Traits and actions such as these describe the complexity leader, who is self-reflective and relationship-based.

Components of Transformational Leadership

Bass and Riggio (2006) enhanced and expanded on earlier work. Building upon their research, they identified four components of transformational leadership: idealized influence, inspirational motivation, intellectual stimulation, and individual consideration. *Idealized influence* is reflected in the trust and admiration that is engendered and the quality of behaviors that move followers toward identification and emulation. *Inspirational motivation* develops as the leader motivates and inspires with effective communication that transmits meaning and challenge to the work and promotes a shared vision. *Intellectual stimulation* is effected through inviting innovation and creativity. New approaches are encouraged and, especially important, there is no public criticism of ideas or mistakes. *Individual consideration* involves treating each person's needs for achievement and growth through coaching, teaching, mentoring, and effective delegation.

Evidence of complexity leadership principles can be seen in these components, especially with the emphasis on relationships. Diverse opinions and ideas are welcomed and, combined with effective delegation, are qualities found in self-organization. The self-reflective aspects of personal transformational leadership are indicative of complexity leadership as well. The following table illustrates the leadership behaviors for each component and describes the environment generated and the expressed perception of the transformational leader.

COMPONENTS OF TRANSFORMATIONAL LEADERSHIP

COMPONENT	LEADERSHIP BEHAVIORS: WHAT ARE THEY?	LEADERSHIP BEHAVIORS: WHAT WILL WE SEE?	LEADERSHIP BEHAVIORS: WHAT WILL THEY SAY?
Idealized Influence	• Role models • Does the right thing • Willing to take risks • High moral and ethical standards	• Admiration • Respect • Trust/ Reassurance • Collective sense of mission	"My leader instills pride in me and specifies the importance of having a strong sense of purpose."
Inspirational Motivation	• Motivates/ Inspires • Imparts meaning and challenge • Charismatic • Optimistic/ Enthusiastic	• Team spirit • Compelling mission • Followers want to meet the challenges • Commitment to meeting goals	"My leader articulates a compelling vision for the future."
Intellectual Stimulation	• Stimulates efforts • Encourages new approaches • Questions assumptions • Reframes problems	• Creativity and innovation are encouraged • There is no public criticism • Anyone at any level or position feels free to contribute ideas	"My leader seeks differing perspectives when solving problems."
Individualized Consideration	• Coach/mentor/ teacher • Recognizes and accepts individual differences • Delegates effectively	• Supportive climate for growth • Personalized attention • Truly listens	"My leader spends time teaching and coaching."

Adapted from Bass & Riggio, 2006.

SITUATIONAL LEADERSHIP

Leadership has been viewed as exercising power by molding organizational environments and managerial control. The next generation of leadership theory was focused on oppositional leadership styles, such as authoritarian versus democratic, and concern for production versus concern for people. Situational leadership, originated by Hershey and Blanchard (1982), was based on several earlier models. These models have characteristics of strategic choice, in that it is the leader who chooses the style and action designed to change the behavior of the employee.

Hershey and Blanchard focused on the two opposing leadership actions of task and relationship. The manager diagnoses the level of maturity in relation to job performance of an individual or group in order to use the best leadership style for a particular situation. Maturity is an individual's willingness and/or ability to do a task at hand. Willingness and ability are influenced by experience, education, and motivation.

Beck and Yeager, in *The Leader's Window* (1994), named their work the L4 system, with the two opposing leadership approaches being direction and support. These correspond with four leadership styles represented as styles 1, 2 ,3, and 4:

1. High direction, low support
2. High direction and support
3. Low direction, high support
4. Low direction, low support

Figure 5-2 illustrates the Leader's Window. Beck and Yeager enrich their model by detailing behaviors that correspond with each leadership style. These are decision-making, communication, and recognition. Table 5–1 details the styles, their ineffective opposites, and the sub-behaviors. Also see *A Case for Complexity* on page 85.

Figure 5-2 The Leader's Window. (Adapted from Beck, J., & Yeager, N. [1994]. *The leader's window: Mastering the four styles of leadership to build high performing teams.* New York: John Wiley & Sons, Inc.)

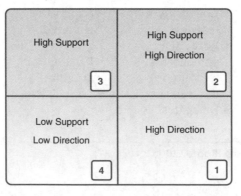

Table 5–1 **LEADERSHIP CHARACTERISTICS**

	STYLE 1: HIGH DIRECTION	STYLE 2: HIGH SUPPORT, HIGH DIRECTION	STYLE 3: HIGH SUPPORT	STYLE 4: LOW SUPPORT LOW DIRECTION
Effective at	Directing	Problem solving	Developing	Delegating
Ineffective at	Dominating	Over-involving	Over-accommodating	Abdicating
Decision making	Leader decides alone	Leader decides with input	Members decide with support	Members decide alone
Communication	Active influencing	Active influencing Active listening	Active listening	Limited influencing Limited listening
Recognition giver for	Complying with orders	Providing input for decision making	Seeking accepting support and guidance	Assuming responsibility successfully

Adapted from Beck & Yeager, 1994.

INFLUENTIAL LEADERSHIP AUTHORS OF THE 1980s AND 1990s

Peters, Hammer, Champy, Block, Handy, and Weisbord influenced management practices and thinking about leadership and came closer to a complexity process. Tom Peters (1982) sounded a shrill bugle in the early 1980s. The hierarchical command-and-control organization and the "stuffy, rigid" business schools that fed and maintained these organizations could no longer sleep after Peters' reveille. He then concentrated on managing the corporation better, followed by teaching how to respond to rapid change and competition. His framework, by his own admission, still glorified big corporate organizations but urged leaders to be less mechanistic.

In *Thriving on Chaos* (1987) Peters proposed moving toward a fundamental dismantling of current structures far beyond hierarchy to concepts like *horizontal, self-contained work teams,* and *networks.* He believed that changing the structure would liberate people to be able to respond to change and competition more readily. He clearly saw restructure (toward less structure) as the answer to creating the new, more organic, entity (Peters, 1992).

As an example of an organization utilizing the new decentralized, more organic leadership style, Peters described the restructuring of Florida's Lakeland Regional Medical Center into a patient-focused care model using care pairs and self-contained work teams.

Peters's guiding principles show the influence of new science/chaos theory. Peters's first three principles are: pursue fast-paced innovation, empower people, and create total customer responsiveness. The fourth principle, especially, represents complexity concepts (Goldberg, Notkin, and Dutcher, 1995): adapt new forms or organization through mastering paradox, learning to live flexibly, and embracing change. This includes:

- Decimating middle-management ranks and demolishing functional barriers
- Structuring the system to the problem (necessary disorganization)
- Leveraging knowledge (information is your product, whatever you make)
- Making every person a businessperson

Although he does not use complexity terms, Peters promotes the practices of complexity leadership. He alludes to chaos theory and his interest in new science in *Liberation Management* (1992), which is subtitled, *Necessary Disorganization for the Nanosecond Nineties.* He reflects that chaos theory "certifies the notion dear to my heart—that the messy aspects of phenomena are the most important" (p. 480). Peters's earlier work, entitled *Thriving on Chaos* (1987), was responding to the macro-level imperative to be part of a management revolution within a chaotic

A CASE FOR COMPLEXITY

Greta, an accomplished clinical nurse specialist, worked in a very busy community hospital psychiatric department. She consulted to all disciplines, taught in-service programs, facilitated research, and provided advanced patient care. She was at a Level 4 according to situational leadership theory. Greta required and asked for very little direction and, while her interpersonal skills were exceptional, she did not have a need for a large amount of attention to relationship. When a position to move into management opened, Greta applied.

David, the department's director, selected her from the pool of candidates because of the respect she engendered, while realizing that she would have a learning curve. David could see that, for the early part of her tenure in the new position, Greta would be at a Level 2, where she needed both increased attention to relationship and some specific direction to learn the human resources and financial aspects involved in health-care management. David reserved the conference room for a 3-hour block. He brought all the financial statements, explanations of variance, and policies and procedures related to managing the budget. David and Greta went through the material, David explaining, Greta asking for clarification. When she was uncertain, he gave her encouragement. When they finished, Greta was feeling better educated but knew she would need ongoing guidance, which David offered readily. He looked forward to seeing her move into Level 3 as she matured in the job, and he fully expected Greta to regain her Level 4 status with experience and support.

economic environment. He writes about a world turned upside down, pursuing fast-paced innovation empowering people for flexibility and learning to love change. Of special focus was his attention to paradox and how important it is for leaders to master paradox. The core paradox for leaders is the need to foster internal stability in order to encourage the pursuit of constant change. Other paradoxes especially in line with complexity thinking are:

- High quality yields lower costs.
- Tighter control can be achieved through more decentralization.
- More appropriate measurement is achieved with fewer measures.
- Success comes to those who love chaos—constant change—not those who attempt to eliminate it.

Peters was embracing complexity concepts such as paradox and complex adaptive systems characteristics of distributed leadership, simple rules, surprise and unpredictability, nonlinearity, and self-organization.

ORGANIZATIONAL RESTRUCTURE

Restructure, often called re-engineering, was the theme of the 1990s and very prevalent in health-care organizations. All organizational structure and business processes are examined to radically change the way work is done and by whom. The hallmark was a change from functional departments to process teams. The business processes drive changes in jobs as well as structures, management, measurement, values, and culture. Hammer and Champy (1993) suggested that all these structural changes were vital to re-engineering. The assumption, as with Peters, is if you change the structure, the people will change. Health-care executives throughout the 1990s eagerly used Hammer and Champy's approach in their restructure projects. Many of these efforts in health care did not last. It can be inferred that structural change without the attention to people in relationships will not sustain long-term progress.

The structure focus was modified and humanized in Peter Block's (1993) concept of stewardship. He, too, flattens the organization and advocates redistribution of power, including abandoning most staff positions and departments and incorporating the work into team functions. Block's emphasis on partnership, service, and abolishment of a class system blends restructure and relationships in a fashion very applicable to health-care systems.

Economist Charles Handy (1995) pushed readers to realize how fast their world is changing, capturing the organizational change trends: "One sign of the new type of organization is a perceptible change in the language we use to talk about organizations. Organizations used to be perceived as gigantic pieces of engineering, with largely interchangeable human parts. We talked of their structure and their systems, of inputs and outputs, of control devices and managing them, as if the whole was one large factory. Today the language is not that of engineering but of politics, with talk of culture and networks, of teams and coalitions, of influence of power rather than control, of leadership not management. It is as if we had suddenly woken up to the fact that organizations were made up of people" (p. 89).

Organizational transformation requires a vision and goals initiated and embraced by large numbers of people in the organization. Weisbord (1992) contributed unique tools for organizational growth and change through his method of conducting future search conferences. Large numbers of players are brought together to achieve shared vision and collaborative action through guided activities and dialogue. The future search generates common purpose, spirit, and empowered action. In health care, where so many people are educated professionals who await recognition as full participants, a future search conference can uncover new levels of learning and commitment. It can be inferred that Weisbord sees people and relationships as the propagators of their own change. The people then bring forth the changes in systems and structures needed to fulfill their vision. Organizations must shift and shift again to grow continuously from within the complexity of relationships, just as individuals change from within.

Outside in, top down, and imposed transformation is an oxymoron. Individuals lead organizations through their interactions with others. These relationships are the seedbed for change. Care must be exercised not to impose new structure in an effort to motivate people to change. The most effective and alive organizations are created when leaders throughout the organization share a vision, information is available in abundance, and all are invited to participate.

The dominant themes that emerge from the management literature in the 1980s and 1990s are:

- Transformational leadership is an effective leadership style.
- Decentralized, point-of-service–driven, people-oriented organizations with empowered self-directed teams are preferable for organizational change.
- Structural change is necessary in organizations for greater productivity and quality.

Although these are effective strategies, standing alone, they demonstrate old-style, mechanistic paradigms and lead to the following assumptions:

- Adopt transformational leadership traits, and the organization can be changed.
- Empowerment, clear direction, and common goals will make high-performing teams.
- Change the structure, and the people will change.

To complete the contextual framework for complexity leadership, whole systems concepts are important. People are self-organizing systems, evolving toward complexity and order and connected in such a way that everyone is a participant. There are no impartial observers. The previous assumptions can then be reframed:

- Transformational leaders are in reciprocal relationships with the system and are transformed by the system's actions and relationships. There are leaders everywhere in the system.
- Empowered, high-performing teams are about relationships and the quality of the interactions among the participants. The relationships at the point of service influence the outcomes of the whole system.
- People in relationships will change the structure, not the other way around.

The health-care environment is one of high drama every day, and it is unpredictable. One severe trauma brought to the emergency room can have a trigger (butterfly) effect that cascades throughout almost every department and discipline in a hospital. Adding to this unpredictability is the pressure of regulatory agencies requiring precise fulfillment of standards.

The urge to have some control and order is understandable. It is difficult to realize and accept that the nature of a care-giving service organization is to be unpredictable and in flux. Care giving does not need top-down control because its true nature must be allowed to emerge. The true nature of health care is a workforce of highly knowledgeable and educated clinicians and operations personnel who, with sound competencies, can make informed decisions at the point of service without referring to others in higher authority.

SUMMARY

There have been multiple influences on the practice of management and leadership over a 100-year span, from workers as rule-following parts of a mechanical operation to independent agents in relationship for distributed control. For leaders themselves, the transition was extremely significant because it brought leaders from outside the system imposing direction to being within the system in relationship with others. Chapter 6 discusses contemporary leadership models and theorists that contribute to an understanding of leadership in the age of complexity.

QUESTIONS FOR SELF-REFLECTION

1. In a health-care organization with which you are familiar, where along the leadership century timeline do you believe the predominate leadership approach falls? Describe your reasoning.
2. How can situational leadership models be helpful in coaching for leadership? Explain.
3. In a restructure, reorganization, or major project in which you were involved, what leadership approaches were used? Were they effective or not? Explain.
4. Do you and the team with whom you work engage in double-loop learning or single-loop learning? What has been the result?

Self-Reflection: What Have I Learned?

_____

_____

_____

_____

_____

5–1 CRITICAL THINKING QUESTION ▰▰▰▰▰

Senge describes several learning disabilities that can occur with a group or team. Review these. How can each of these be modified or corrected by employing complexity thinking? Write an exemplar that either illustrates some of these myths in action or how the opposite, not buying into the myths, has proved successful.

5–2 CRITICAL THINKING CASE
FOR COMPLEXITY ▰▰▰▰▰

I was recently asked to assume the role of interim nurse manager, in addition to my role as clinical nurse educator, on a 23-bed mother-baby unit in a tertiary academic medical center. Over the years, it has been a personal frustration to see what I perceived as a lack of engagement in professional development by the nursing staff. As an advocate of lifelong learning and higher education, I am surprised by the number of nurses who do not pursue higher education, membership in their professional specialty organization, or membership on nursing committees. I feel it is important that nurses stay informed. Personally, new knowledge and ideas drive my desire for professional growth and clinical excellence. It confused me to think others might not have the same goals.

The mother-infant unit (MIU) is a complex adaptive system embedded in an academic medical center. Within the MIU are patients, families, and employees from a variety of ethnic, cultural, economic, and educational backgrounds. The National Database of Nursing Quality Indicators survey results for the unit reveal overall high job satisfaction scores, with the lowest score related to involvement with hospital affairs.

For the most part, nurses contribute little to their annual performance appraisal. Goals and objectives are discussed at the time of the appraisal, and self-evaluations have not been used. Due to union membership, nurses' rate of pay and raises are based on the hospital's agreement with the union and not on merit. There are no clinical ladders or professional growth incentives.

As the interim nurse manager, I viewed my role as temporary. Subconsciously, I must have believed I should just stay the course and keep the ship from crashing or sinking while waiting for the former nurse manager to return or for a new captain to take the ship. While attending a nursing leadership course in which participants explored the concept of complexity science, I had an epiphany. I have been going with the status quo, accepting the linear model of leadership in my work environment. The single most important idea that I took away from the course is that one small action can have a large impact. I have decided that when I return to work, I will change course, take a risk, and prepare to navigate new waters, even if they are a little rough.

After reflection, I thought that perhaps my goal of higher education for all is not a shared goal, nor does it need to be. The goals for the unit are high-quality patient care, patient satisfaction, and staff satisfaction. Maybe we can get there without every nurse setting a goal for higher education. With reflection, I also realized that the nurses have not been well supported to participate in professional development. Often, implementation of policies, procedures, and practices comes from the top down. Staff input may be requested but, if not forthcoming, there are no creative attempts to elicit ideas.

My intention is to share some of the concepts I learned in the course and to lay the foundation for a more caring, self-aware work environment. I feel I have gained a new view of my unit and the hospital by seeing things through the lens of complexity. The principles I will use as a foundation include: building a good enough vision, leading with clockware and swarmware in tandem, and tuning into the edge on the unit. My tool kit will include the use of generative relationships, minimum specifications, simple rules, and reflection. Nurses will be asked to reflect on questions and share ideas. Self-reflection will be encouraged before annual performance appraisals, with the nurse's insights and goals included in the evaluation.

My vision is that by demonstrating and promoting caring, appreciative inquiry and encouraging reflection , staff and patients will feel cared for. I imagine I will hear, "What happened to Debbie? The new leader looks like her, but something happened to her at that course she took last summer!" But I will know that I am well on my way with my journey from linear to complexity leadership.

5–3 CRITICAL THINKING QUESTION ▬▬▬

Reflect on your work environment. Using your complexity lens, describe what you see and how you would move it further away from linear and toward complexity.

REFERENCES

Argyris, C. (1991). Teaching smart people to learn. *Harvard Business Rev, 4*(2), 4-14.

Bass, B.M., & Riggio, R.E. (2006). *Transformational leadership* (2nd ed.). Mahway, NJ: Lawrence Erbaum Associates.

Beck, J., & Yeager, N. (1994). *The leader's window: Mastering the four styles of leadership to build high performing teams.* New York: John Wiley & Sons.

Block, P. (1993). *Stewardship: Choosing service over self-interest.* San Francisco: Berrett Koehler.

Burns, J.M. (1978). *Leadership.* New York: Harper & Row.

Dunham-Taylor, J. (1995). Identifying the best in nurse executive leadership. *J Nurs Adm, 25*(7/8), 24-31.

Gardner, H. (1995). *Leading minds: An anatomy of leadership.* San Francisco: Basic Books.

Goldberg, E., Notkin, D., & Dutcher, R.F. (1995). *The Tom Peters business school in a box*. New York: Alfred A. Knopf.

Hammer, M., & Champy, J. (1993). *Reengineering the corporation*. New York: Harper Business.

Handy, C. (1995). *The age of paradox*. Boston: Harvard Business School Press.

Hershey, P., & Blanchard, K. (1982). *Management of organizational behavior utilizing human resources* (4th ed.). Englewood Cliffs, NJ: Prentice-Hall.

Marquis, B., & Huston, C. (2000). *Leadership roles and management functions in nursing*. Philadelphia: Lippincott Williams & Wilkins.

Marriner-Tomey, A. (1993). *Transformational leadership in nursing*. St Louis: Mosby–Year Book.

Peters, T. (1992). *Liberation management*. New York: Harper and Row.

Peters, T. (1987). *Thriving on chaos*. New York: Alfred A. Knopf.

Peters, T., & Waterman, R. (1982). *In search of excellence*. New York: Warner Books.

Senge, P.M. (1990). *The fifth discipline: The art & practice of the learning organization*. New York: Doubleday/Currency.

Stacey, R.D. (2003). *Strategic management and organisational dynamics*. Harlow, United Kingdom: Pearson Education.

Swanberg, R., & Swanberg, R. (2002). *Introduction to management and leadership for nurse managers* (3rd ed.). Sudbury, MA: Jones & Bartlett Learning.

Watzlawick, P., Weakland, J., & Fisch, R. (1974). *Change principles of problem formation and problem resolution*. New York: W.W. Norton & Co.

Weisbord, M. (1992) *Discovering common ground*. San Francisco: Berrett Koehler.

6

CONTEMPORARY LEADERSHIP MODELS THAT REFLECT COMPLEXITY

The complexity leader is embedded in the system, not in control, but with a complexity view and simple rules creates the environment where relationships thrive and people self-organize.

■ OBJECTIVES

- Discuss leadership research and models related to complexity science.
- Apply complexity-inspired leadership theories and models to contemporary health-care practice.
- Assess personal leadership qualities and behaviors.
- Analyze leadership models and theories in relationship to the Complexity Leadership Model.

INTRODUCTION

Leadership styles and personal leadership qualities are presented in this chapter. Helgesen's (1995) *Web of Inclusion* was one of the first to describe leadership that entailed an organizational approach that represented complex adaptive system thinking. Microsystems leadership behavior is also based on the complexity premise. The leadership models *stages of personal power in organizations* (Hagberg, 1984) and *Level 5 leadership* (Collins, 2005) provide an opportunity to assess one's qualities of leadership. The role of emotional intelligence (Goleman, 1998) in effective leadership contributes understanding of the importance of personal self-reflective, relationship-based leadership. Porter-O'Grady and Malloch (2007) describe the leader in a complex system as one who is vulnerable and willing to participate in the cycle of vulnerability.

A look at the phenomenon of control for complexity leaders is discussed as well. Johansen proposes leadership skills that will be needed for the volatile, uncertain, complex, and ambiguous world of the future.

THE WEB OF INCLUSION

One of the first authors to study and write about new science leadership was Sally Helgesen. While interviewing female leaders for her book, *The Female Advantage* (1990), she discovered a leadership style distinctly different from a top-down hierarchical structure. These leaders were embedded in the system, surrounded by others, always in communication, with very little focus on titles or roles (Fig. 6-1). She investigated this phenomenon further. The result was her second work, *The Web of Inclusion* (1995). The organizations she studied had broken away from the top-down mode to a more organic, "leader in the center" practice, which Helgesen termed a *dynamic connectedness*.

The web is both pattern and process. The pattern resembles a web, with the leader in the center and many connections across and up and down the structure. There is flexibility and, as an open system, roles and responsibilities change as needed; thus, new lines of relationships develop over time. There is less reliance on titles, perks, and symbols, with a more collegial atmosphere in its place. Information flows freely across lines, an example of Stacey's systems parameters of flow of information. The web by its very nature includes more people at all levels in decision making, in contrast with hierarchical structures, which are by nature more exclusive. Helgesen offers six characteristics of webs in operation (Box 6–1), illustrating the web as process.

1. *Open communication across levels:* Information is free-flowing. Neither good nor bad news is held back.

Figure 6-1 An inclusive leadership style.

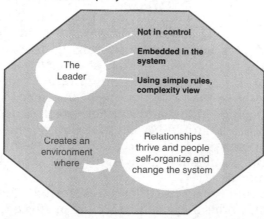

Box 6–1	HELGESEN'S WEB AS PROCESS

- Open communication at all levels
- Blurred distinctions between conception and execution
- Creation of lasting networks that redistribute power
- Serves as a vehicle of constant reorganization
- Embraces the world outside the organization
- Evolves through a process of trial and error

From Helgesen, 1995/2005.

2. *Blurred distinctions between conception and execution:* There is less division between those who plan and decide what will be done and those who implement the ideas.
3. *Creation of lasting networks that redistribute power:* Once people come together for a project, they keep these relationships going, forming alliances and connections both formal and informal that help their work going forward.
4. *Serves as a vehicle for constant reorganization:* New connections between and among people and permeable boundaries create conditions for evolution to new improved ways of doing the work.
5. *The world outside the organization is embraced:* There is a conscious effort to reach out to customers and community outside the organization.
6. *Evolution through a process of trial and error:* Diffuse decision-making power at local levels of the organization and freedom to try new things are encouraged and supported.

Helgesen discusses several challenges to becoming a weblike organization: marketing, diversity, empowering the front line, making training part of the process, and building strategic alliances. She contends that everyone should be viewed as a marketer rather than keeping marketing as a separate stand-alone department. If people think as marketers, they will be looking for ways to improve the product to meet a need. Respecting and encouraging diverse opinions and perspectives is the natural consequence of a web. New technology and new ways of working require that those in the front lines or at the point of service have the power to make the needed decisions and innovations. Ongoing training and learning for all in order to seek ways to constantly improve should be part of the work, not separate. Partnerships are necessary in a fast-paced world. As technology helps organizations become smaller, organizations need to reach out to others for mutual support.

One organization Helgesen studied was Boston's Beth Israel Nursing Department, under the vice presidency of Joyce Clifford, and its phenomenally successful primary nursing model. The partnership between Clifford and the CEO Mitchell Rabin demonstrated exemplary leadership. The Beth Israel model was a web, with distributed power and decision making at the point of service. Nurses were encouraged and supported to coordinate care and work with other disciplines to provide care at the bedside. This web had evolved over 25 years, and those who were there at the time of Helgesen's study still express a high level of pride and excitement at being a part of such a dynamic, ever-improving, empowering organization. Unfortunately, a merger with another hospital was a huge clash of cultures, from which the Beth Israel web never fully recovered (Weinberg, 2003). However, it can be rightfully said that the ideas and experience of that era have been transmitted throughout nursing and health care and can be recognized in, for example, Magnet organizations.

STAGES OF PERSONAL POWER

One's way of being a leader is the product of personal and professional development. To transform organizations from top-down, command-and-control entities to organic, self-organizing systems requires leaders whose style is congruent with the latter. Hagberg (1984), in *Real Power,* delved into the behaviors of people in relationship to personal power. She defines personal power as "the extent to which one is able to link the outer capacity for action (external power) with the inner capacity for reflection (internal power)" (p. xvii). Hagberg considers personal power as developmental (Box 6–2). One must grow from stage to stage. She believes that people actually experience and describe power differently in each stage. A review of the six stages follows.

- Stage 1 persons are powerless. They manipulate. They are insecure and dependent, low in self-esteem, uninformed, and helpless. Fear often prevents them from advancing to the next stages.
- Stage 2 persons see power by association. They emulate their superiors, believing them to have a kind of magic. While learning the ropes in the organization, they are dependent on their supervisor. They experience a new self-awareness and feel stuck about moving. The need for security may hold them back.
- Stage 3 persons interpret symbols as signs of power. They strive for control. They are egocentric, realistic, competitive, expert, ambitious, and often charismatic. Not knowing they are stuck can hold them back. Many leaders fall into this stage.
- Stage 4 persons come to understand power through intense self-reflection. They have genuine influence. They are competent, strong, comfortable with their personal style, and skilled at mentoring and show true leadership. They may not move ahead if they fail to let go of their egos. Helgesen sees these as the most admired in most organizations.

Box 6–2	HAGBERG'S STAGES OF PERSONAL POWER

Stage 1: Powerless
Stage 2: Association
Stage 3: Symbols
Stage 4: Self-reflection
Stage 5: Purpose
Stage 6: Wisdom

―――――――――

From Hagberg, 1984/2003.

- Stage 5 persons experience power because they are confident of a life purpose beyond themselves. They have vision. They are self-accepting, calm, humble, and generous in empowering others. A lack of faith can keep them from reaching the next level.
- Stage 6 persons see the whole picture. They are wise. They are comfortable with paradox, unafraid of death, quiet in service, ethical, and do not have the need to feel powerful. They see and feel things on the universal plane. Only human constraints can hold these people back. They usually do not seek leadership positions when at this stage.

Stage 3 and 4 leaders constitute the majority of leaders in all organizations, including health care. External organizational rewards are important to Stage 3 people, which are provided by the typical health-care environment. Symbols of status are abundant in hospitals. The line between exempt positions and hourly positions is heavily drawn, even though many of the hourly employees are professional clinicians with college degrees. Perhaps senior management's concern with perks, office location, and titles of authority can be attributed to the need to emulate corporate business as much as possible and to compensate for salaries that are much lower in hospital systems than in large corporations. It is not unusual to find a small-to-medium community hospital with eight to ten vice-presidents and three to four layers of directors and managers below that.

Porter-O'Grady and Wilson (1995) call for dismantling this hierarchy to three levels of management, at most, with two levels being even more desirable. They propose that vice-president roles should be removed, with the supporting departments, such as finance, human resources, and operations, given service or consulting role definitions and titles. All work should be organized around patient care point-of-service with front-line, point-of-care managers having the skill and knowledge that in the past was held by vice presidents. There should be few barriers from community to board, from chief executive officer to the entire system. All departments should be horizontally integrated. "Relationships, not status, define value" (p. 118). Stage 3 leaders cannot deliver the leadership for this new health-care system described by Porter-O'Grady and Wilson.

A person who answers "yes" to the following sample questions most likely identifies with Stage 3:

1. Do you feel that you have to prove yourself because you have been given responsibility?
2. Do you think that power is finite, that there is only so much power to go around?
3. Are symbols extremely important to you, like salary, title, material possessions, office placement, or number of supervisees?
4. Do you believe power means being in control of others?

Hagberg describes Stage 3 as predominantly masculine, with traits such as egocentric, realistic, competitive, expert, ambitious, and charismatic. While the symbol for this stage is status, the operative power word is control. Many successful leaders have been and are Stage 3, loving the symbols of their success and achievements and accepting that control is the best way to lead for productivity and adherence to standards. A classic manifestation of this in health-care systems is the proclivity for writing new policies and procedures. These are often written to correct one identified problem or error. Frequently, quality assurance indicators are used solely to monitor performance and to catch people doing something wrong.

Women have more difficulty with Stage 3 and are more comfortable with Stages 2 and 5. Most feel that Stage 3 behaviors conflict with their natures, which are generally more comfortable with relationships and shared power. Generally, success in an organization entails working at Stage 3 while establishing a place in the organization and in acquiring recognition.

Women on senior management teams who have been clinical practitioners, where there are both feminine and caring orientations, may experience conflict with the predominant Stage 3 leadership of others in the group. Learning the ways of Stage 3 without giving up one's own style is desirable (see *A Case for Complexity*). Often, women nurse executives have taken on the role of Stage 3 leadership in order to fit in and, in some cases, survive. This can cause severe cognitive dissonance for them when it conflicts with their values and also alienates them from their clinical colleagues, who perceive them as having sold out. Cognitive dissonance is a state of psychological discomfort because of inconsistencies in cognition such as conflict between current conditions, how one behaves, and what one values (Festinger, 1957). The case for everyone to develop Stage 4 leadership can be seen clearly as a way to reconcile the dilemma. Stage 4 leaders most likely identify with the following questions:

1. Do you feel as if you have a life going on inside of you that is distinctly different from the one on the outside?

A CASE FOR COMPLEXITY

As health-care systems launch, restructure, and redesign patient care projects, a phenomenon is surfacing where the chief executive officer (CEO) and other senior leaders may be at Stage 3 while the directors, supervisors, and clinicians are operating at Stage 4 (quadrant 3 in the linear/complexity matrix). For example, a hospital's CEO daringly undertook the restructure of the entire hospital to patient-focused care primarily to reduce spending, but he also envisioned himself to be the leader of the first community hospital in the region to change the entire organization (including outpatient services). Status was important to him as he sought for this recognition and prestige. Fortunately, the clinical managers creatively embraced the new plans, and a talented education department supported their efforts, and real transformation occurred.

At a progress meeting that included the CEO, vice presidents, and other managers, the facilitator was encouraging stories of success from those areas already practicing in the new way. One director was describing how well patient room and bed assignments were going now that the administrative support associates had been upgraded and trained to coordinate unit activities. Previously, registered nurses (RNs) would be pulled from the bedside, and everything would stop while the room/bed assignment was made by the RN. This held up the patient and family (usually in the hallway) as well as the operating room or emergency department transportation person. As the director was relating this, the CEO became visibly anxious and interrupted, "but where is the control? Shouldn't someone in higher authority, like the RN, make that decision?" The Stage 4 (and some Stage 5) leaders present, with the facilitator's help, quickly explained the beauty of the success, and fortunately the CEO listened and perhaps was nudged a little closer to Stage 4 himself.

2. Is it important for you to have a natural and personal style that is yours and not what the organization expects?
3. Have you had a major crisis or triggering event in your life that has challenged the way you think about life and work?
4. Do you find that the symbols of success do not flatter or motivate you the way they used to?
5. Do you acknowledge both feminine and masculine behavior as useful, depending on the situation, and use them appropriately?

Hagberg (1984) describes her Stage 4 leader as having power by self-reflection. The traits of Stage 4 include being competent, reflective, strong, and comfortable with one's own style and being skilled at mentoring

The transition from Stage 3 to 4 is about self-development and requires considerable effort. Development from Stage 1 to 2 is externally motivated; changing from Stage 4 to 6 involves internal growth. Leaving behind the predictable concrete expectations of Stage 3 and becoming more self-reflective and aware is the challenge to striving for complexity leadership. The ultimate goal for complexity leaders is to move forward into Stage 5, where personal being and awareness support their quest.

Hagberg encourages those who wish to develop to Stage 5, Power by Purpose, to become less attached to status and ego in order to model the traits of self-acceptance, calmness, having vision, humility, having a life purpose, and being generous in their empowerment of others. Spirituality is developed and displayed in Stage 5. Knowledge of self, commitment to serve, vision, and being an educator, communicator, and comforter describe a leader who is conscious of relationships and connections, what Greenleaf (1977) called servanthood. Stage 5 leaders tend to identify with the following questions:

1. Are you comfortable enough with yourself that other people's opinions of you do not affect you?
2. Do you have a life purpose that reaches beyond yourself and your organization?
3. Do you have a deep inner core of spirituality?
4. Do you operate out of a quiet, inner sense of calm?
5. Is your ego getting smaller and less significant all the time?
6. Do you consciously give power away by empowering others?
7. Do you feel your work and your life are becoming more integrated, less splintered?

The characteristics of Stage 6 leaders include their comfort with paradox and being unafraid of death. They are powerless, meaning they need very little tangible power. Quiet in service and ethical, they often seem to live on a universal plane, with a larger understanding of the world. Although Hagberg believes that Stage 6 leaders have no need to be leaders or seek powerful positions, one can wonder if complexity leaders would do well with (and be expected to have) some Stage 6 traits. The questions for Stage 6 follow, but be aware that Hagberg embeds irony there, and she even adds that it is a trick quiz, a true paradox. If you think you are Stage 6, then you probably aren't!

1. Do you see all of life as paradox?
2. Do you understand the interrelationship of all things?
3. Is service to the world of individuals "your work"?
4. Do you operate on an inner set of ethical principles that pervades your life?

5. Are you committed yet detached?
6. Are you unafraid of death?
7. Do you frequently ask unanswerable questions?
8. Do you have a life purpose for which you would die?
9. Do you feel complete peace of mind?
10. Are you considered a sage?
11. Do you enjoy long periods of solitude and silence?
12. Are you nearly perfect?

THE ROLE OF EMOTIONAL INTELLIGENCE IN EFFECTIVE LEADERSHIP

In his 1998 article in *Harvard Business Review,* Daniel Goleman built upon his book *Emotional Intelligence* (1994) to relate the qualities of effective leadership). As part of a review of leadership competencies models, Goleman evaluated 188 companies. When he calculated the ratio of technical skill, IQ, and emotional intelligence, emotional intelligence was given twice as much importance as the other two. While this was true for all levels of the organizations, the higher the level of the leader, the more that emotional intelligence was an indicator of success.

The five components of emotional intelligence are self-awareness, self-regulation, motivation, empathy, and social skill. The first three are about self-management, and the other two are about managing relationships. Table 6–1 lists these characteristics with their definitions and hallmarks.

These five components can be found within the complexity leadership model. Empathy and social skill are essential elements of a transformational leadership style. Self-awareness and self-regulation are integral to personal being and awareness. Motivation is the desire to achieve rather than just acting from external rewards. It is the very trait needed to take action as a complexity leader. It is acting beyond expectations with intense commitment and high standards. In Unit Three, Personal Being and Awareness, there is more discussion of emotional intelligence.

LEADERSHIP IN MICROSYSTEMS

Successful microsystems attribute their effectiveness to an active process of leadership. The 20 microsystems studied by Batalden et al. (2003) revealed three core processes to active leading that contributed to the performance of the units. These are building knowledge, taking action, and reviewing and reflecting.

Building knowledge involves learning everything about the basic structure, process, and pattern of the microsystem. Knowing as much

Table 6–1	COMPONENTS OF EMOTIONAL INTELLIGENCE	
COMPONENENT	**DEFINITION**	**HALLMARKS**
Self-awareness	Recognizing your moods, emotions, and drives and their effect on others	Self-confidence with realistic self-assessment and self-deprecating humor
Self-regulation	Controlling/ redirecting disruptive impulses and moods, suspending judgment, thinking before acting	Trustworthy, comfortable with ambiguity, and open to change
Motivation	Working with passion, not just for money or status, with energy and persistence	Driven to achieve and committed to the work; optimistic even in the face of failure
Empathy	Understanding the emotional makeup of others and treating people according to their emotional reaction	Builds and retains talent, cross-culturally sensitive, service-oriented
Social skill	Managing relationships through networks; finding common ground and building rapport	Leads change effectively, persuasive and expert team builder and leader

From Goleman, 1995.

as possible means measuring, monitoring, and noticing the work process to see what can be changed. It entails being open to others' feedback about what works and what does not and to new ideas for change and improvement.

Taking action involves the leader being "in the midst," actively engaged in the daily workings of the microsystem. Creating the most effective reporting relationships and technology as well as work-flow methods for cooperative functioning of the whole group requires an active participating leader.

Reviewing and reflecting means setting the tone and creating the structure for the groups to reflect on their goals, vision, and the effects of changes that have been made. Leaders create the time and space for earnest review and reflection on the microsystem's patterns of practice. They are creating the space for double-loop learning as well.

Another leadership practice common to successful microsystems is the absence of a single, lone leader. Instead, consistently across the studied microsystems, there were two or three co-leaders; partnerships; some combination of physicians, nurses, and administrators. These interdisciplinary connections exemplify the relationship aspects of successful complex adaptive systems.

LEVEL 5 LEADERSHIP

In *Good to Great* (2001), Collins reports on a 5-year study of 28 successful companies. Although the researchers deliberately did not focus on the executives, the experience of the team and the data pointed out strongly that there was a pattern that could not be ignored. The successful companies all had leaders with common characteristics, a combination of modesty, willfulness, humbleness, and fearlessness. Collins terms this the highest level of leadership in a hierarchy of five levels (Fig. 6-2). The Level 5 leaders were distinguished by a paradoxical blend of humility and professional will. They were self-effacing, always putting the success of the company first.

Collins delineates the five levels as (1) highly capable individual, (2) contributing team member (3) competent manager (4) effective leader and (5) Level 5 executive. The Level 5 leaders were much more interested in their companies' long-term prospects than their own reputation for personal greatness.

Many leaders attain Level 4, but Collins maintains that the move from Level 4 to 5 is not easily accomplished. A "seed" within these leaders determines the platform for Level 5. Their egos get out of the way for something larger than themselves. The seed may sprout through self-reflection or a profound transforming event that brings these leaders beyond their own self-service.

An interesting discovery made by the team was a phenomenon termed the window and the mirror effect. When contrasting Level 5 leaders with others, the team indicated that Level 5 leaders looked out of the window to give credit to others when things went well and into the mirror to take responsibility when things went wrong. They often attributed success to good luck, not themselves. The less successful (not Level 5) executives reversed the window and mirror analogy. They credited themselves for achievements and blamed others, not themselves, for unsuccessful outcomes.

The question remains whether leaders can learn to become Level 5 leaders. One of the issues is that Level 4 leaders are often seen as the

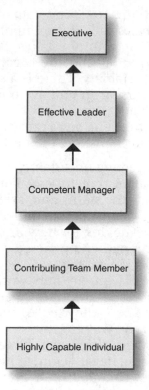

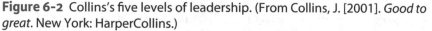

Figure 6-2 Collins's five levels of leadership. (From Collins, J. [2001]. *Good to great*. New York: HarperCollins.)

prototype of great leaders: vigorous, visionary, and visible. Achieving Level 4 is an accomplishment in itself, but those qualities that include more concern for fame, fortune, adulation, and power are not in keeping with Level 5 leaders. Collins hypothesizes that for some, the Level 5 seed is simply not there. Those with the seed may evolve under the right circumstances, either through intense self-reflection or a life-transforming experience. Inner development is the key.

LEADERSHIP VULNERABILITY

Porter-O'Grady and Malloch (2007) discuss vulnerability as a key component needed to lead in a quantum organization. A quantum organization is one in which the leaders embrace complexity and concepts of the new science. They hold to the new view that openness— to others and to new ideas—is positive leadership vulnerability. Vulnerability is present when leaders are able "to examine long held beliefs and change their minds without feelings of inadequacy, recognize personal limitations and strengths, and work from a clearly defined personal identity" (p. 167). The vulnerable leader is not weak or incompetent but creates an environment for safe and healthy dialogue and is not afraid to admit mistakes. Leadership vulnerability sets the stage for each person and the organization as a whole to embrace the cycle of vulnerability. There is a six-step process, a cycle of vulnerability, that occurs again and again as a leader is willing to learn to live in vulnerability (Box 6–3). The six steps are: becoming vulnerable, taking risks, stretching one's capacity, living the new reality, evaluating the results, and cherishing the new knowledge gained.

- *Becoming vulnerable:* Accepting uncertainty, tolerating discomfort, admitting fallibility, making time for creativity
- *Taking risks:* Challenging the status quo, asking the unaskable, encouraging tinkering, being open to difficult issues
- *Stretching one's capacity:* Looking for new untapped potential, sharing uncertainty, strengthening sacred connection, creating conditions that support risk taking
- *Living the new reality:* Allowing the new work to be integrated into the system, being ready for unanticipated outcomes, coaching to sustain the new knowledge, encouraging others to be vulnerable, leading the way to trust
- *Evaluating the results:* Measuring beyond linear cause and effect; acknowledging and using negative outcomes to learn, correct, apologize, reassess the goal, modify, or even abandoning if necessary
- *Cherishing the new knowledge gained:* Making use of what was learned about what worked and what did not to help with future projects

THE ILLUSION OF CONTROL

One commonality in all of these approaches to leadership is the willingness to let go of control. Planning and control efforts reduce anxiety and bring some stability, but they stifle creativity as well.

Box 6–3   LEADERSHIP VULNERABILITY CYCLE

Becoming Vulnerable
   Taking Risks
      Stretching One's Capacity
         Living the New Reality
            Evaluating the Results
               Cherishing the New Knowledge

From Porter-O'Grady & Malloch, 2007.

Complexity leaders are comfortable with uncertainty, and they are open to self-organization. They have made the choice between two competing mental models. The first is that health-care organizations are bureaucratic, tightly managed, well-oiled machines where bottom-line and aligned incentives are paramount. The contrasting mental model has surprise and uncertainty as opportunities, and the best ideas often come from the edge or the shadow system (Anderson and McDaniel, 2000; Olson and Eoyang, 2001). Whether leaders are in the middle of Helgesen's web or microsystem; comfortable with ambiguity, or empowering and attributing success to others, they recognize the illusion of control and willingly let it go. Johansen (2012) incorporates the concept of control in the elucidation of his 10 leadership skills for the future. Control is illusionary, and leaders need skills that take into account accelerating disruptive change or VUCA: volatility, uncertainty, complexity, and ambiguity. Johansen is articulating the essence of a complex adaptive system, such as our health-care organizations. Furthermore, the skills correspond to the main concepts in complexity leadership to a great extent. Both are based on viewing the world and organizations from a complexity perspective. The 10 skills are described below with commentary about the relationship to complexity leadership concepts.

1. *Maker instinct*: The ability to use inner drive to build and grow an organization. Nurses inherently use this skill when pursuing the best care for their patients.
2. *Clarity:* Being able to see through the present difficulty with a larger view, projecting a clear goal but giving others the flexibility to take the steps to achieve the goal in a distributed leadership fashion.
3. *Dilemma flipping*: Not easily solved, dilemmas have an element of paradox in them that requires a leader who can turn these into opportunities and advantages.
4. *Immersive learning ability*: Immersing oneself in situations and conditions that promote learning, the ability to be embedded, in the midst of the complex adaptive system
5. *Bio-empathy*: Seeing the organization and culture from the perspective of nature, acknowledging that self-organization, interconnectedness, and complexity are the way the world works.
6. *Constructive depolarization*: The ability to relate to people on all sides and to calm tense situations, hallmarks of personal being and awareness.
7. *Quiet transparency*: Being open and authentic, not self-promoting, developed through the practice of personal being and awareness.
8. *Rapid prototyping*: Not waiting to develop a product or try an intervention until there is perfection, but being willing to learn from first attempts, as in improving clinical interventions

based on just-in-time discovery rather than data analysis months after the data is collected.

9. *Smart-mob organizing:* Effective communication both in person and with electronic media, essential skills for every day and into the future

10. *Commons creating*: The ability to work with others to nurture shared assets, creating a balance of cooperation and competition as is seen in complex adaptive systems; this skill builds upon the nine others.

SUMMARY

There are leadership models in contemporary practice that exemplify complexity. These models illustrate the need for transformational, self-reflective, relationship-based behaviors. The leader is deep within the system, not outside and observing it. The focus is on relationship building, not role definition (Anderson and McDaniel, 2000). Begun and White (2008) capture this: "A complexity inspired approach to leadership recognizes that the future is unknowable and unpredictable but that its emerging features are shaped by those individuals and organizations with the competencies to explore, connect, and make sense" (p. 256). In Chapter 7, models and practices of organizational culture and change are presented. This is essential knowledge for the complexity leader.

QUESTIONS FOR SELF-REFLECTION

1. With what stage of personal power do you most identify? Explain.
2. Review emotional intelligence leadership traits. Where do you believe you are in failing to achieve these behaviors?
3. How web-like is the organization in which you work or one with which you are familiar? Describe your observations.
4. How is the issue of control played out in your organization? What is your tendency in regards to being in control?

Self-Reflection: What Have I Learned?

_____

_____

_____

_____

_____

6–1 CRITICAL THINKING EXERCISE ▬▬▬

Review the leadership models in this chapter. Choose two to compare and contrast. Then explain how these models exemplify complexity science concepts.

6–2 CRITICAL THINKING CASE
FOR COMPLEXITY ▬▬▬

I was appointed coordinator of an associate degree nursing program that provided the first 2 years of nursing education in what was actually a 2+2 design. The program was unique in that students could complete their associate degree in 2 years as opposed to many programs offered by community colleges, which required that prerequisites be met before entry into the nursing component of the program. I began this new administrative role in the fall of the year that our NCLEX pass rate plummeted from 90% the previous year to 63%. As the faculty began to examine many components of the program, as well as admission criteria, I met with the president of the university's student nurse organization. She was concerned about the success of her classmates on the upcoming licensing exam the following spring and was campaigning for an NCLEX review course, which we had never offered on campus. This discussion spurred me to look at supplemental programs being offered by several vendors to provide standardized testing throughout the program, followed by an NCLEX review course. I had been in favor of adding this type of service in past years, but my colleagues had not been convinced of the merits of such a program.

I invited vendors to campus to meet with faculty and introduce their product, which resulted in the selection of a program that offered comprehensive testing, remediation, and a review course, at a reasonable cost to the students. The problem was that I wanted to start right away, but I had not built the fees into the budget for the current year. I had to convince the chair of the department, faculty members, and students that this was a worthwhile investment and get the students to agree to pay for the spring semester themselves. Faculty agreed to move forward; the chair of the department offered to cover a portion of the fee for the students; and after meeting with each group of students and highlighting the advantages of adding this program, all the students paid their share of the semester fee. In the spring semester, we embarked on the integration of standardized testing and more intensive NCLEX preparation as part of a comprehensive plan designed to improve student outcomes on the licensing exam. These efforts resulted in an increase in board scores that first year to 73% and further integration of standardized testing into the curriculum along with other changes over the next few years.

The cost of student participation in a supplemental program has been built into the lab fees following that first-semester campaign. This was a change that has been sustained and improved upon, and 3 years later the first-time pass rate for our graduates was 89%. We recently switched to a different vendor, and another faculty member serves as administrator of the supplemental testing program for our department, but the tenets of this value-added service remain solid.

6–3 QUESTIONS FOR CRITICAL THINKING AND DISCUSSION

From a complex adaptive system's perspective, who were the various constituencies involved and what mental models might they have held?

This coordinator describes her experience in a matter-of-fact manner, which belies her leadership skills. In complexity science terms, describe what characteristics of complexity leadership she exhibited and what skills and behaviors helped her to implement the new program?

REFERENCES

Anderson, R.A., & McDaniel, R.R. (2000). Managing health care organizations: Where professionalism meets complexity science. *Health Care Manage Rev, 25*(1), 83-92.

Batalden, P.B., Nelson, E.C., Mohr, J.J., et al. (2003). Microsystems in health care: Part 5: How leaders are leading. *Jt Comm J Qual Saf, 29*(6), 297-308.

Begun, J., & White, K. (2008). The challenge of change: Inspiring leadership. In C. Lindberg, S. Nash, & C. Lindberg (eds.), *On the edge: Nursing in the age of complexity*. Scotts Valley, CA: CreateSpace.

Collins, J. (2001). *Good to great*. New York: HarperCollins.

Collins, J. (2005). Level 5 leadership: The triumph of humility and fierce resolve. *Harvard Business Rev*, July/August, p. 1-12.

Festinger, L. (1957). *A theory of cognitive dissonance*. Stanford, CA: Stanford University Press.

Goleman, D. (1995). *Emotional intelligence*. New York: Bantam Books.

Goleman, D. (1998). What makes a leader? *Harvard Business Review*, November/December, pp. 93-102.

Greenleaf, R. (1977/2002). *Servant leadership: A journey into the nature of legitimate power and greatness*. New York: Paulist Press.

Hagberg, J.O. (1984/2003). *Real power: Stages of personal power in organizations* (3rd ed.). Salem, WI: Sheffield.

Helgesen, S. (1990). *The female advantage: Women's ways of leadership*. New York: Doubleday Currency.

Helgesen, S. (1995/2005) *The web of inclusion*. Frederick, MD: Beard Books.

Johansen, B. (2012). *Leaders make the future: Ten new leadership skills for an uncertain world* (2nd ed.). San Francisco: Berrett-Koehler.

Olson, E.E., & Eoyang, G.H. (2001). *Facilitating organizational change: Lessons from complexity science*. San Francisco: Jossey-Bass.

Porter-O' Grady, T., & Malloch, K. (2007) *Quantum leadership*. Sudbury, MA: Jones & Bartlett Learning.

Porter O' Grady, T., & Wilson, C. (1995) *The leadership revolution in health care*. Aspen Publications.

Weinberg, D.B. (2003). *Code green: Money driven hospitals and the dismantling of nursing*. Ithaca, NY: Cornell University Press.

7

ESSENTIAL KNOWLEDGE
FOR COMPLEXITY LEADERS

Leap from stone to stone when crossing a rushing stream. Be nimble.
Scan for the next best step; then leap. That is the complexity leader way.

■ OBJECTIVES

- Assess organizational culture through examination of artifacts, espoused values, and shared underlying assumptions.
- Apply the concepts of positive deviance to complex adaptive systems.
- Compare and contrast the role of the change agent in culture and change theories.
- Analyze selected change theories within the framework of complexity thinking.

INTRODUCTION

Culture and change are natural aspects of living and of the life of organizations, and they are the focus of this chapter. With awareness and understanding of these elements, one can develop a true complexity perspective, a way to think about organizations that is essential for successful complexity leaders. Assessing the overall culture helps leaders discover what is going on in the system. This enables the leader to be a better change agent. Peter Vaill, organizational management consultant and author, introduced the concept of *permanent whitewater* to describe rapid, chaotic change. He defines permanent whitewater as a "continual succession of surprising, novel, ill-structured, and messy events, which force themselves on a manager's attention and which as an ongoing kind of disruptive event cannot be planned out of existence"(Olsen and Eoyang, 2001, p. xxix). Vaill reflects that until his exposure to complexity thinking, he did not have a frame for how he could work productively within "the midst of the swirl." Schein's organizational culture model is seminal and applicable to understanding health-care organizations. Three change theory models are presented. (1) Roger's diffusion of innovations is becoming a classic and continues to provide insight into how people and organizations adopt and adapt to change initiatives and interventions, such as new technology or practices. (2) The complex adaptive model of organizational change fully embraces the complexity perspective into a very workable model for leaders who want to be agents of change. (3) Positive deviance is helping communities and systems move toward making improvements. The success of a national effort to reduce methicillin-resistant *Staphylococcus aureus* (MRSA) infection rates using positive deviance is an exciting example of complexity science concepts in action.

ORGANIZATIONAL CULTURE

Schein (1992) sees leadership as creating and managing the organizational culture. An organizational culture includes behavior, common values, group norms, language, philosophy, habits, mental models, and climate. Schein brings these concepts together for his definition of organizational culture, which is: "a pattern of shared basic assumptions that the group learned as it solved its problems. The pattern has worked well enough to be considered valid and, therefore, to be taught to new members as the correct way to perceive, think, and feel in relation to those problems" (p. 12).

Schein states in his latest work on culture "I will continue to argue (1) that leaders as entrepreneurs are the main architects of culture, (2) that after cultures are formed, they influence what kind of leadership is possible, and (3) that if elements of the culture become dysfunctional, leadership can and must do something to speed up culture change" (Schein, 2010). Analyzing culture entails assessing the levels of culture. The process moves from the obvious or tangible artifacts, to the deeper espoused values, to the deepest underlying basic assumptions, or the essence, of the culture. Artifacts are easy to see but hard to decipher. They are the visible organizational structures and processes, what one sees walking through the door. In addition to the physical aspects of architecture, there are the products, style of dress, manner of interacting, and even emotions, stories, rituals, and routines. While obvious, their meaning is not always clear. An organization's culture can be misperceived because one's own interpretation and values may get in the way. A person who values an orderly work atmosphere may enter a busy, chaotic-looking nursing unit and think that nursing care is not very good without really knowing whether that is so.

Going deeper reveals the culture's espoused values. These are the values and beliefs about what works and what does not work, usually arrived at by social validation of the group. People together have the same experiences and create meaning. Values are the strategies, goals, and philosophies of the group. At the conscious level, the group subscribes to moral/ethical rules and beliefs as members work to keep uncertainty and anxiety in their place. The espoused values may be what people in the group say that they believe, but the people may not actually act within their stated values. For example, a hospital may say that it is very patient-focused and that it puts patients' needs first, but it may have a rigid visiting policy that contradicts that value.

The deeper level to probe is that of basic underlying assumptions. It is here that true culture is revealed. Basic underlying assumptions are unconscious beliefs, thoughts, and feelings of the group and culture. They are the ultimate source of values and action and often are taken for granted. These assumptions are rarely confronted or debated, and thus they are hard to change. People want to perceive the events around them as congruent with their assumptions. Schein (1992) refers to this inclination as a psychological defense mechanism. One individual's assumptions may be more easily challenged than a group's, which are so much more entrenched. All the efforts to improve the quality of care in hospitals, such as the work of the Institute of Medicine or the Institute of Healthcare Improvement (IHI), are difficult because of underlying assumptions. For example, one provider may assume it owns the health-care organization and that patients should just do as they are told. Donald Berwick of IHI (2004) remarks, however, that providers should be viewed as guests in the patients' lives instead. If the underlying assumptions are not discerned, then it will be hard to decipher the artifacts or determine if the espoused values are credible. Changing a culture when seen from this perspective can be difficult, time-consuming, and anxiety-provoking.

The ultimate goal for a healthy culture is the alignment of what is seen (artifacts), what is said (espoused values), and what is believed (underlying basic assumptions). See Fig. 7-1. The purpose of assessing

Figure 7-1 Understanding an organization's culture.

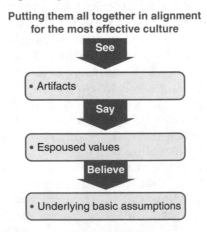

Putting them all together in alignment
for the most effective culture

See

• Artifacts

Say

• Espoused values

Believe

• Underlying basic assumptions

a culture is usually to understand it. For example, assessing is essential for a new leader when entering the organizational culture. But more often the goal is to change the culture or a portion of it. This may be driven by internal conflict or outside stress to improve. It always requires a leader, a facilitator, or an informal leader who recognizes the need to identify issues and work for change. Time and space are needed to bring people together for dialogue and reflection.

HOW LEADERS CREATE OR CHANGE ORGANIZATIONAL CULTURE

Before change can be attempted, it is important to know the organization's culture. This is best done through helping the organization understand its own culture. There are several assumptions to be aware of when starting this process. Because culture is a set of shared assumptions, work with the group, not individuals. Also, it is more valuable for the group to understand its culture than for the outsider. Focus on the portion of the culture that is affected by the issue to be solved or the change to be made. Trying to change an entire organization's culture can take upwards of 3 years, a massive undertaking. An outside facilitator is needed to help all the groups uncover their assumptions. This can be someone from the education department who has credibility with the group or an independent consultant. The uncovered assumptions usually fall into one of two categories: those that help resolve issues or further strategic goals, and those that hamper or constrain. Having the group sort and identify these assumptions promotes reflection and fosters planning for the future. It may be discovered that the culture in place already can solve the issues and problems by building on existing assumptions.

Before embarking on deciphering cultural assumptions, the leadership must commit to the process. As Schein (1992) cautions, if there is not a reason, an issue, or high interest in finding solutions, the group will not be engaged to any real extent. In a large-meeting format, the first task is for the group to learn about the organizational culture characteristics of artifacts, espoused values, and shared underlying assumptions. The group is helped to identify the artifacts. The group is encouraged to describe the organization: how people dress, behave, use space, keep order, follow routines, address supervisors, and display emotions are a few items to consider. After a substantial list is generated, the group can start to discuss, based on these artifacts, why they do things the way they do. For example, a hospital may have a very plain lobby with outdated furniture. When asked why, they may say it is because they put their money into patient care, or that they see no need to impress people.

When a list of values and beliefs has been generated, the group can turn to underlying shared assumptions. How congruent are the artifacts and the expressed values (beliefs)? Referring to the previous example, the group may discover during discussion that little importance is placed on creating a pleasant environment for patients, families, or even themselves. Perhaps for this group it stems from an austere approach originated by certain founders that just continued. The group may be sharing an underlying assumption that paying attention to the attractiveness of the work space for themselves and the caring space for their patients is frivolous. One of the reasons for even convening the group may have been an issue of losing market share to the new clinic in town (after having no competition). With help, the group may see that the assumption may be holding it back from attracting or keeping patients and that, at a deeper level, not enough attention has been paid to creating a healing environment for patients. In this case the artifacts, expressed values, and shared underlying assumptions might be congruent, but they do not serve the patients, the group, or the viability of the hospital.

Schein compares this work of helping with culture identification and organizational change with Lewin's three stages of the change process: unfreezing, movement, and refreezing (Tiffany and Lutjens, 1997). Discovering the shared underlying assumptions (Table 7–1) is stage one, Lewin's unfreezing, as the group comes to realize through reflection what lies below the surface of work. As the group

Table 7–1	**SHARED DISCOVERY OF ORGANIZATIONAL CULTURE**	
ARTIFACTS	**ESPOUSED VALUES**	**SHARED UNDERLYING ASSUMPTIONS**
What is going on here? What is it that we do?	Why do we do it? What does it mean?	What do we really believe and assume?
Dress-code behavior Use of time Use of space Methods of communication How supervisors are addressed	How do we explain our artifacts, our everyday practices? What do we say are our values that inform our work practices?	Do our espoused values really explain our artifacts? Is there a disconnect? If so, what assumptions about our work are really in effect?

Adapted from Schein, 1992.

makes these discoveries, people are then open to making changes by either changing some of their assumptions or building upon those that are useful to their change process. Then they can confirm and solidify their new way of thinking and behaving—refreezing. However, people who view organizations as complex adaptive systems now believe that it is almost impossible to attempt a refreezing because constant change and adaptation are ever present in successful organizations.

ESTABLISHING A LEARNING CULTURE

Building on concepts from the learning organization, Schein (1992) proposes characteristics of the learning culture. A learning culture contains a core assumption that organizations can manage and adapt to their environments. Another core assumption is that people can be proactive problem solvers and learners. Regarding the nature of reality and truth, the learning culture is pragmatic rather than moralistic and authoritative. It is naturally able to change. Groups and individuals with a balance between authority and collegiality form the best relationships. In a turbulent environment, it is best to think far enough ahead to assess consequences yet focus near enough to see what is working. Being fully connected through information and communication is another hallmark of the learning culture. An orientation to the work and leadership that is both relationship- and task-oriented promotes learning. Finally, moving away from linear thinking toward systemic thinking will enhance the learning culture. Complexity thinking emphasizes relationships, groups coming together to discover their shared meaning, and being ever-adaptable to the changing landscape. There is a reinforcement of less emphasis on control by the leader.

CHANGE THEORIES AND COMPLEX ADAPTIVE SYSTEMS

Change theories play a large role in understanding and leading health-care organizations. Roger's diffusion of innovations continues to develop and intersect with complexity concepts. Olsen and Eyong's change approach is based on complexity science concepts and the role of the change agent within the complex system. Finally, positive deviance has demonstrated its applicability to solve behavioral, social, and health-care problems and is decidedly illustrative of complexity principles in practice.

Rogers's Diffusion of Innovation

Rogers's diffusion of innovations explains the process of change and how a new concept or innovation takes hold and spreads throughout a system. The focus is on an individual or a group and the learning process in deciding whether to adopt an innovation. There is uncertainty and perceived risk involved in the diffusion process. The diffusion of new ideas is described as an "innovation that is communicated through certain channels over time among members of a social system" (Rogers, 2003, p. 36). Rogers's change works when put into play and encompasses culture and communication as well as conflict. Figure 7-2 presents Rogers's Diffusion of Innovations Model.

An innovation is an idea, practice, or object that is perceived as new. The innovation has five attributes through which it is viewed by perspective adopters: the relative advantage, compatibility, complexity, trial-ability, and observability. These five attributes influence the interest and acceptance of the innovation. Messages about the innovation may be person to person, group to group, or mass media. Communication is more easily accomplished when the group is alike (homophily) rather than diverse (heterophilous), where people are less alike in thought and values and, therefore, the conflicts that arise cause change and acceptance to be more difficult. The time required to diffuse an innovation is described by Rogers as steps and rate. There is a sequence, a process that leads to adoption. First, there is knowledge (awareness) of the innovation. Then an attitude develops, which can lead to acceptance or rejection. The persuasion step is where one is persuaded to accept the innovation.

Figure 7-2 A model of five stages in the innovation-decision process. (Reprinted with the permission of Free Press, a Division of Simon & Schuster, Inc., from DIFFUSION OF INNOVATIONS, 5th Edition by Everett M. Rogers: Copyright © 1995, 2003 by Everett M. Rogers. Copyright © 1962, 1971, 1983 by The Free Press. All rights reserved.)

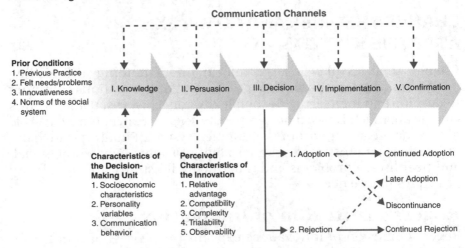

The next three steps are decision (to accept or reject), acceptance, and implementation and confirmation. The rate at which the innovation is diffused throughout the system is based on the response of different people in the system. There are the innovators, the early adopters, the early majority, late majority, and finally the laggards, who may never adopt at all. Table 7–2 describes the categories of adopters and their distribution in a given system based upon extensive innovation research.

The social system in which innovation takes place is a set of interrelated units that join together to solve problems and work toward solutions with common goals. There is structure and patterns that facilitate or impede the diffusion. The established behavior patterns form norms that influence how people in the system relate to and adapt to change. The change agent attempts to influence others' decisions to adopt the innovation. There are also change aids that, although not having formal roles, may help with the diffusion by widely coming into contact with others to influence them. Of much importance to an innovation's success are opinion leaders who have enormous influence and usually fall into the early adopter category. They are the true champions for the initiative and are essential for a leader—the change agent—to accomplish the effort. The change agent may use different methods to promote the decision to adopt the innovation. Sometimes a person decides to adopt independently of others; this is the optional style. A collective type of decision requires consensus, whereas an authoritarian method uses the power of authority, status, or technical expertise. A leader might use a combination of two methods, which Rogers terms contingency. When the social system is considering whether to adopt an innovation, the consequences for doing so are usually considered. For example, during the United States national heath-care reform conversation, many people were for "reform" until they started to consider the consequences and how it would affect their own health care.

Stages of Diffusion and the Role of the Change Agent

In the knowledge stage, people tend to expose themselves to experiences and new ideas that are in keeping with their own ideas and attitudes. They will see a need or be made aware. They will seek information to reduce the anxiety of not knowing so they can fulfill that need. If they hear that a new technology is on the market and it is important to them to have the latest, they will seek information. The least difficult people are those who already have a mindset for that new idea. Leaders as change agents can create the need by first creating awareness that the new item exists and then offering information about how it will

Table 7–2   ADOPTER CATEGORIES, DISTRIBUTION, AND CHARACTERISTICS

INNOVATORS	EARLY ADOPTERS	EARLY MAJORITY	LATE MAJORITY	LAGGARDS
2.5 %	13.5%	34%	34%	16%
VENTURESOME	RESPECTED	DELIBERATE	SKEPTICAL	TRADITIONAL
• Rash, daring • Has complex knowledge • Can cope with uncertainty • Has financial resources • Gatekeeper for new ideas	• Local person • Opinion leader • Role model • Gives stamp of approval	• Follower • Deliberate • Willing but seldom leads	• Cautious • Adopts because of system and peer pressure • Must feel safe	• Past is point of reference • Suspicious of change agents • Holds traditional values • Usually has fewer resources

Adapted from Rogers, 2003.

help them. Rogers believes that not all early "knowers" turn into early adopters. Some of the facilitators for this are education, the structure of the system, mass media, interpersonal channels, amount of contact with the change agent, how others in the system are participating in the change, and how cosmopolitan (connecting with others outside of the bounds of the systems) the knowers are. All these can be influenced by the leader as the change agent. Notice how these facilitators involve relationships with others, the leaders, peers, and with people and ideas outside of the immediate system.

The persuasion stage is mostly about feeling and attitude as opposed to the knowledge stage, which is cognitively based. The individuals form attitudes and consider change as they become more active and involved. They seek information and ask, "What is in this for me?" It is interesting that attitude and action may be different. Often people believe and agree that some healthy living habits—such as not smoking or overeating—are good, but they do not follow through with action to change. Health-care workers know that consistent hand washing is of utmost importance in reducing infections, but they may be inconsistent with their own hand-washing routine. Rogers refers to this as the "KAP gap" (knowledge, attitude, practice). A cue to action can help change the behavior. This is an event that can crystallize a favorable attitude toward the change. If a person witnesses a friend or relative go through an experience that could have been prevented, such as not getting a mammogram and then developing cancer, this solidifies the attitude, and the behavior is changed. A cue to action may be internally driven, as just described, or it can be offered, as in incentives or rewards. Additionally, for hand washing, plotting and posting infection rates on patient care units for all to see may serve that purpose. Occasionally, negative events, such as a poor Joint Commission score, can be very effective in changing practice. There are opportunities for change agents to employ cues to action to further the persuasion stage.

In the decision stage, people choose to adopt or reject the innovation. They may try it, see a peer use it, or have it demonstrated to them. Demonstration can be quite effective. The process usually follows the stages in order—knowledge, persuasion, and decision. In an authoritarian setting, people may go right from knowledge to decision and skip the persuasion stage altogether. There are several ways that people reject an innovation. They may be aware and then "forget." They may adopt and then discontinue. They also may actively reject by considering and then rejecting or, in a passive manner, never considering it in the first place.

In the implementation stage, the innovation is put to use, and there is overt behavior change. There may still be uncertainty, as when working with new technology. With organizations it can be harder to effect the behavior change because the system itself may obstruct the process. There are so many elements in the system—formal structures, policy, and procedures—that strive to maintain the old order and stability. Implementation contains within it a good bit of reinvention, especially in an effective organization. Continuous change and adaptation are accepted, and people are open to change and improvement in the system. There may be passive adaptors who think things should stay the same after the change is made, and then there are active modifiers who understand that different individuals and organizations require modification over time. Assuming that the innovation can be the same individual to individual or organization to organization implies that all individuals and cultures are the same and is a false notion. Reinvention actually facilitates the rate of adoption and sustains it going forward.

An innovation is not a fixed entity. Contrary to change theory that suggests the change should be fixed, adopters are open to more change. "Potential adopters often can be active participants in the adoption and diffusion process, struggling to give meaning to the new idea as the innovation is applied to their local context" (Rogers, 2003, p. 187). This description of reinvention reflects the complex adaptive system's view of organizations as self-organizing, with local agents contributing to system changes.

The confirmation stage occurs when people are presented with the innovation as they seek to diminish cognitive dissonance between their knowledge and attitudes and actual behavior to continue the new practice. Some people, however, discontinue the new practice, rejecting after first adopting. They either replace it with something better or, because of dissatisfaction, decide to stop. They may not see the relative advantage, or the innovation has not been fully integrated into their work or system. Later adopters are more likely to discontinue the adopted practices. There are many implications for change agents to employ leadership that facilitates the other stages—knowledge, persuasion, and decision—for longer-term acceptance.

Change Agents as Linkers

Change agents facilitate the flow of innovation but must be careful not to overload the system with excessive information, which can cause a breakdown in the initiative. The more that the norm in the organization is one favorable to change, the easier it is to facilitate an innovation. Seven sequenced roles for the change agent are suggested by Rogers:

- Develop a need for change awareness.
- Establish information exchange relationships and rapport.
- Diagnose problems but be empathic to others' perspective.
- Create an intent to change.
- Translate intent into action.

- Stabilize the adoption and prevent discontinuance.
- Achieve a terminal relationship—local agents can self-renew and not depend on the change agent.

There are factors that contribute to the change agent's success. The change agent needs to devote much time and energy to contact and communication, requesting and accepting feedback, with a real emphasis on others' needs. This is similar to Batalden's (2003) use of attractors as motivators and the importance of selecting these attractors based on what the staff considers motivators, not what the leader wants. Empathy is essential for engaging others and determining what will motivate them. The leader must be seen as having credibility for others to accept the new ideas. It is easier when there is congruence in the thinking and approach and values with those whom one leads (homophily), but the greater challenge is with those who do see things differently (heterophily). Then the true talent and skills of conflict management are called forth.

One of the change agent's most important assets is the opinion leader who can carry the message; this leader is often referred to as the champion for the change. Opinion leaders most often are early adopters. They are frequently found in middle management, close enough to staff to see what is occurring and to be a role model. Characteristics for effective champions include occupying a key linking position, possessing analytical and intuitive skills to understand others' aspirations, and having well-developed interpersonal and negotiating skills. Opinion leaders may not be in top powerful positions, but are adept at handling people. These are all skills called for in complexity leaders. All nurses can be opinion leaders and champions, but advanced practice nurses are in a unique position to do so because of their graduate education and prominent, pivotal roles. Advanced practice nurses in health-care organizations, whether in practice roles or in management, are uniquely positioned to become opinion leaders and champions for innovations and best practices.

Centralization Versus Decentralization

When the theoretical framework for diffusion was developed and then researched worldwide, the underlying assumption was that these innovations would diffuse and take hold within a centralized, top-down system. The researchers discovered that, contrary to this, often the diffusion could and would take hold in decentralized organizations. If there is technical expertise involved or a public health issue for which people see no need, centralizing will work best. But otherwise, decentralized diffusion systems are client-controlled with wide sharing of power and may "bubble up from local experimentation by non-expert users who participate, create, and share information with one another in order to reach a mutual understanding" (Rogers, 2003, p. 401). The researchers were discovering the effectiveness of self-organizing complex adaptive systems.

The Change Agent From a Complexity View

Olson and Eoyang (2001) present a complexity view of facilitating organizational change. They refute the traditional assumptions of organizational change that envision organizations as machines. The traditional assumptions, or truisms, about change are: change starts at the top, efficiency comes from control, and prediction is possible. These organizations are leader-driven and are based on continuous measurement and controlling feedback of people and processes. Furthermore, the leader is expected to calm turbulence while leading a whole systems change. This approach does not work in a self-organizing system.

The complex, adaptive model of organizational change is derived from concepts of self-organization, system's agents, change agent, and patterns. The assumptions are that order is emergent, not hierarchical; the history of the system is irreversible; and the system's future is often unpredictable. The complex adaptive system is composed of agents in the system who are semiautonomous. Change agents are system agents who consciously attempt to influence the self-organization process. They may be from any level, internal or external. Patterns emerge from the self-organizing process, agents interacting in real time. Structure, culture, and behavioral norms are examples of emergent patterns.

Self-organizing dynamics is the process by which the parts of the system—the system agents, ideas, people, departments, and clients—act to generate a whole systemwide pattern (phase 1). Then these emergent patterns, mental models, team, and delivery systems cultures start to affect the parts (phase 2). In phase 1, patterns of everyday ways of working and setting up processes and procedures are established and fine-tuned. However, once the pattern is established, while valuable for keeping actions and decision automatic and for keeping order, the pattern can become entrenched and then hold back change and innovation. This constant interaction keeps the system going, but is "messy and iterative, lurching and searching" (Olson and Eoyang, 2001, p. 11) the way to new organizational structures and relationships.

Conditions for Self-Organization

The change agent, understanding complex adaptive systems and self-organization, can seek to influence the system by using three factors that affect the placement, shape, and power of self-organizing patterns. These are: containers, significant differences, and transforming changes.

- *Containers:* Set the bounds by building organizational-departmental conceptual rules, purpose, procedures, behavior, culture, professional identification

- *Significant differences:* Determine the primary patterns—power, level of expertise, gender, race, educational background—and the differences that affect the work and relationships
- *Transforming exchanges:* Connections between the system's agents, where information and resource vehicles include meetings, e-mail, memos, phone calls, and delivery systems

Containers hold the system together and can be magnet-like, such as a strong leader who draws people in; or fence-like, defining the outside limits of the system; or characterized by affinity as in culture, gender, or discipline that binds the agents in the system. Containers are also the basis for values, norms, and beliefs that contain and constrain the patterns in the system. Each organization has a different set of significant differences that shape the emerging patterns. In health care, for instance, various disciplines have different knowledge, practices, and power. Transforming exchanges connect various systems agents to each other. There can be too little exchange, leaving people feeling isolated and uninformed, or too much information, which feels like micromanagement and stifles creativity and growth.

These factors, which may be observed and assessed separately in the organization by the change agent, are in reality interconnected, and a change in one affects the other two. The change agent understands the evolving patterns and usually selects one condition that may be the easiest to start, makes an intervention, and evaluates the outcome. There may be a shift in the other conditions as a result of the intervention as well.

The Complex Adaptive Model method for the change agent is akin to the nursing process or a quality improvement initiative: assess, set goals, decide on actions, and employ an intervention. The change agent starts with assessing the conditions for self-organization. First, the container is examined to determine how constrained the system is between one that is too strong, with over-firm boundaries and rigidity, and one that is too diffuse and weak. Next the change agent determines the state of the significant differences. Are they hidden and not acknowledged? Are there many and all given the same weight? Are differences that constrain or unconstrain the system acknowledged and then worked through? Are there meaningful transforming exchanges and contact among the agents that form the patterns; are there many, but all top-down; or are there very few and trivial? After assessing to determine the level of self-organization by how under- or over-controlled it is, the change agent can select which of the three areas to target, then set goals and choose actions. Usually the actions taken with one area will start to move the whole in the right direction. The accompanying *A Case for Complexity* describes this process.

The role of the formal leader includes being a change agent. Olson and Eoyang (2001) suggest that the leader set the tone through attending to the container, focusing on significant differences, and facilitating transforming exchanges.

Set the Container
Influence the environment that influences the system by:

- Setting few key expectations, with general requirements for outcomes, and let the agents determine how to proceed
- Distributing control for a pattern of respectful trust
- Generating a sense of urgency that encourages trials and pilots
- Stretching boundaries, using small experiments, assigning new responsibilities and roles
- Shrinking boundaries when necessary to provide constraint if there is information overload or the rate of change is too fast
- Being clear about mission

Focus on Significant Differences
Focus on those that will shape productive patterns. For example:

- Explore contradiction; surface, acknowledge, and resolve tensions
- Accept contention and adversity; conflict signals growth and learning
- Raise tough questions; increase connections, and inspire vision
- Encourage workforce diversity for a lively mix of agent activity
- Understand significant differences in the external environment; scan for innovation by others

A CASE FOR COMPLEXITY

On an acute care nursing unit, the nurse satisfaction scores for the day staff were declining. This seemed to have started the previous June, when five new graduates were hired. At that time, the unit ran smoothly and met benchmarks for patient care outcomes. The nurse manager asked the clinical nurse specialist (CNS) for some help in figuring out what was going on. No one complained to the nurse manager, and she believed she worked hard every day to get the work done, to keep the staff informed, and to advocate for them. The CNS then reviewed the unit and attended some staff meetings. She conducted focus groups and examined the nurse satisfaction data in detail. She discovered that the unit was rule-bound, but not excessively. However, the older, more experienced nurses were the enforcers of the rules over the younger new graduates. There was little conversation between the two groups, other than clinical talk. At staff meetings, the conversation was mostly one way, the nurse manager giving updates, distributing new polices, and providing all the information she believed staff members needed to do their jobs.

A CASE FOR COMPLEXITY—cont'd

Assessing the container as just about right for self-organization, the CNS could see that the significant differences of age and experience of the nurses was not being acknowledged at all or discussed, and the transforming exchanges were almost exclusively top-down. When the experienced nurses were asked why they did not speak at staff meetings, they replied that they had given up long ago. The nurse manager meant well but really did not want to hear from them. They felt they got done what needed to be done clinically very well, and they were the ones who kept the unit running. The new graduates told the CNS that they were too scared to speak up; if the experienced nurses remained silent, the new graduates thought that was the way staff meetings were supposed to run.

The CNS chose to work first on the transforming exchanges; believing that until there was a healthy communication up as well as down and among all the staff, significant differences could not be surfaced and worked through. She related her findings to the nurse manager, who was open to coaching, and then the CNS called on a colleague in the education department. Together they facilitated an afternoon retreat for the unit day staff. They supported the nurse manager in acknowledging the dissatisfaction reflected in the survey data. They employed some safe communication and team-building exercises. The nurse manager asked for help from staff in changing the format of the staff meetings to be inclusive and collegial in nature.

Communication in staff meetings changed, and with support from the CNS, in time the group felt comfortable enough to work through the generation and experience differences, ultimately becoming more appreciative of each other. Six months later, the nurse manager and the CNS reviewed the latest nurse satisfaction data and were pleased with the improvement. The CNS as a change agent had helped the manager to become her own change agent.

Design Transforming Exchanges
Foster co-evolution with linkages between agents. For example:

- Encourage feedback, such as by asking, "How am I doing?"
- Link communities of practice; identify and encourage linkages internally and externally
- Reconfigure (loosen or tighten) networks; maintain balance between too-exclusive tight relationships and little connection
- Encourage learning; promote information flow and personal and professional development

In a complex adaptive system, the complexity leader as a change agent can effect change through connections, adapting to uncertainty, being comfortable with emerging plans and patterns, and not being afraid of differences but amplifying them for real change and growth. The complexity leader sees success as not closing some gap to reach an ideal but seeing change and activity as fitting with the environment. Whether the leaders are attempting to learn about or change a culture, help people employ best practices, or be a change agent for self-organization, approaching with a complex adaptive systems perspective will serve the leader well. One intervention for promoting change in organizations and communities that exemplifies complexity is positive deviance.

POSITIVE DEVIANCE

Positive deviance started as a research tool used in nutritional sciences. Jerry Sternin and his wife Monique took the basic precepts and developed an action tool that they used worldwide to bring about community improvement. The positive deviance approach is not needs- or problem solving–based but seeks to identify and optimize the solutions already existing in the community. As staff for Save the Children, the Sternins were on assignment to reduce malnutrition in children in Vietnam. They discovered that most of the children in the villages were malnourished and some who were not. Upon inquiry, they determined that the mothers of the well-nourished children were feeding them more often and supplementing the usual rice with shrimp, crab, and sweet potato leaves. This food was considered "poor people's food" by most of the villagers. In true positive deviance fashion, the successful mothers were engaged to show and coach the other mothers. In daily meetings, they practiced the new behaviors, and over 80% of the children were adequately nourished as a result (Buscell, 2004).

The essence of positive deviance is that it is not the outside experts but the successful insiders who effect the best changes in practice and behavior. Positive deviance operates contrary to classic change theories, where it is proposed that knowledge changes behavior and that the progression is *first* knowledge, *then* attitude, and *finally* change of practice. Positive deviance turns that around to practice, attitude, and *then* knowledge. The practice changes the attitude; then the knowledge is internalized. Jerry Sternin reflects, "It is easier to act your way into thinking than to think your way into acting" (Buscell, 2004, p. 11). Positive deviance is not for every problem but for those needing social, attitude, and behavior change. It is useful for people who share the same complex system and can adopt the most successful behaviors of their peers. There are technical and knowledge problems where clearly an outside expert is required for changes in practice to occur.

Positive deviance is effective in health-care situations and has been used with asthma and HIV/AIDS patients to help them stick to arduous medication regimens. One area in which positive deviance can be effective is with hand washing in hospitals, and studies are under way. Statistics show that 60% of nurses and other health-care providers and only 30% of physicians consistently wash their hands, even though they know the value for preventing infections. Plexus Institute, with a Robert Wood Johnson foundation grant, is partnering with 40 hospitals nationwide to decrease the prevalence of methicillin-resistant *Staphylococcus aureus* (Buscell, 2006). Six beta sites are applying three prevention guidelines. The first is to identify at least one target unit for very active surveillance, such as nasal swabs and appropriate isolation. They have agreed to use positive deviance as the approach to finding solutions that already exist in the hospital. All data will be submitted to the National Health Care Safety Network, a Web-based program operated by the Centers for Disease Control and Prevention. In participating hospitals, small solutions by the hundreds have been implemented. These solutions have often been contributed by maintenance, housekeeping, radiology, or physical therapy. The positive deviance focus on increasing prevention compliance is a process of a group transforming their culture from within. One of the leaders remarked: "The closer the staff is to the solution, the more effective and durable these solutions are. In addition to working better and being more self-sustaining, solutions that are created by the staff tend to be simpler and less expensive than those that are mandated or come from outside consultants" (Buscell, 2004, p. 13).

Positive deviance is distributed leadership, with changes in practice that occur at the local level in a self-organizing manner. The characteristics of positive deviance are similar to those of a complex adaptive system, embedded in the culture, generative, building on self, and based on strengths. A leader who facilitates positive deviance is in the role of searcher and inquirer, inviting stories, listening more than talking, allowing the group to bring the solutions, and letting go of control because the people are the experts. With positive deviance, leaders are encouraged to consider approaching change management by taking on a role different than top down. "Managers overlook the isolated successes under their noses or, having appropriated them, re-package the discoveries as templates and disseminate them from the top. This seldom generates enthusiasm necessary to create change" (Pascale and Sternin, 2005, p.1).

Leaders can discover the positive deviants, the innovators who are the key to change. Positive deviance puts leaders in different roles: expert becomes learner, teacher becomes student, and leader becomes follower. The leader in positive deviance is not a path-breaker, but an inquirer, not problem-focused but a discoverer of solutions already embedded in the system. The difference between traditional leadership and positive deviance includes the moves from outside to inside, from deficit-based to asset-based, and from problem identification to solution discovery (Pascale and Sternin, 2005).

SUMMARY

Wheatley and Kellner-Rogers write in *A Simpler Way* (1996) that when organizations are considered as people in relationships, able to create systems and solutions, the people can be nourished with information and be trusted to self-organize. The lesson from complex adaptive systems is that new structures emerge from relationships. When the situation is complex and new thinking is needed, two or more people coming together, each with an idea, will create something better than any one could accomplish alone. Schein's view of organizational culture, Rogers's description of diffusion throughout a complex system, Olson and Eoyang's complex adaptive model, and positive deviance process all exemplify complexity and are essential knowledge for the complexity leader. In Chapter 8, interventions related to communication and teams are addressed.

QUESTIONS FOR SELF-REFLECTION

1. Imagine yourself as a stranger to your organization. When walking through the front door, what artifacts do you see?
2. Into which adopter category do you fall? How does this play out in your work and life?
3. How are significant differences handled in your organization?

Self-Reflection: What Have I Learned?

_____

_____

_____

_____

_____

_____

7–1 CRITICAL THINKING CASE FOR COMPLEXITY

When working as a clinical specialist for a patient monitoring company, I observed the introduction of changes to nursing work flow resulting from new technology. I was responsible for following up with customers after they had their new equipment for 3 to

4 months. On occasion, there were satisfaction issues with a customer that required more immediate attention.

On one occasion, I was notified that the nurses in a community hospital emergency department (ED) were refusing to use the newly installed central station and were quite vocal with their complaints. Before my scheduled visit, the only information I received was that they were refusing to use it and felt all it did was add noise to an already noisy environment.

When I arrived in the ED, I was received rather coolly by the first two nurses that I met. Luckily the ED was rather quiet, with only two non-monitored patients who needed little attention. It was a somewhat small unit with only eight monitored beds. The nurse's station was rather small, enclosed in glass, and had one central monitor and one recorder with a stream of paper hanging from it onto the floor. When I approached the door to the nurse's station, Margaret, a nurse, blocked the door and said, "I'm *not* going to use a mouse, and you can't make me!" The other nurses just ignored me.

"How about a trackball?" I asked, "Would you use a trackball?"

"What's a trackball?" she replied.

I called the biomedical technician clinical educator contact I had for this hospital, and I was informed I would have a trackball in about a half hour. This gave me some time to find out what the nurses' issues were with the new central monitor.

Margaret needed little encouragement to tell me about the events leading up to the central station installation and voice her complaints about the system. About 8 months earlier, a patient had died. The patient was on the bedside monitor, but the alarm volume was turned low. The patient had a fatal dysrhythmia, and no one heard the alarm in the busy, noisy ED. As a result of this incident, risk management and the nurse manager had decided to purchase a central station. This would allow central monitoring of the eight beds, and they thought it would prevent a similar event in the future.

When the clinical educator from my company had the training classes for the nurses, only about 15 of the 44 nurses attended. Two of the nurses were designated "super users" and were responsible for training the other nurses. Most of the nurses still did not have any training, and one of the super users was out on medical leave. Of course, the fact was that the nurses really did not care if they were trained or not, but they knew it was their responsibility to be competent with all equipment in the ED.

A few of the other nurses joined Margaret for a complaint session. I listened to all of their issues and concerns: the alarm noise, the constant recorder paper flow, and so on. I offered to review the features and functionality with them, focusing on the issues they had identified. After I checked the configuration of their system, I asked if their manager would be able to discuss some possible changes. When she arrived, she and the nursing staff described their work flow. I made a few recommendations for changes to the central station configuration that would reduce the number of non–life-threatening dysrhythmia alarms. I told them ways of further reducing alarms by adjusting alarm limits as appropriate for the patient and turning off dysrhythmia alarms that were not appropriate, e.g., the irregular heart rate alarm for the patient in atrial fibrillation.

I split the 10 nurses into three groups and did a review of the central station with each group, having Margaret use the trackball. It turns out that she actually liked it. She said that it was easier to use than the mouse and that it did not require as much space in the nurses' station. I focused on only the capabilities that would affect their work flow. When I showed the full disclosure application to view all the waveforms, the nurse who had cared for the patient who had died said, "If we'd had this equipment, not only would we have been aware of the alarm, but we also would have been able to see the patient's condition leading up to the alarm." The installed help application was also well received. They were able to see the value of the additional technology in their workspace.

7–2 QUESTIONS FOR CRITICAL THINKING AND DISCUSSION ■■■■■■■

Choose one of the models in this chapter to apply to this case for complexity.

REFERENCES

Batalden, P.B., Nelson, E.C., Mohr, J.J., et al. (2003). Microsystems in health care: Part 5. How leaders are leading. *Jt Comm J Qual Safety, 29*(6), 297-308.

Berwick, D.M. (2004). *Escape fire: Designs for the future of healthcare.* San Francisco: Jossey-Bass.

Buscell, P. (2006). Plexus versus the bacteria. *Emerging,* Winter, pp. 1-24 (Plexus Institute, Bordentown, NJ).

Buscell, P. (2004). The power of positive deviance. *Emerging,* August-September, pp. 8-15 (Plexus Institute, Bordentown, NJ).

Heider, J. (1986/2005). *The tao of leadership.* New York: Bantam Books.

Olson, E.E., & Eoyang, G.H. (2001). *Facilitating organizational change: Lessons from complexity science.* San Francisco: Jossey-Bass.

Pascale, R.T., & Sternin, J (2005) Your company's secret change agents. *Harvard Business Review,* May, pp. 1-13.

Rogers, E.M. (2003). *Diffusion of innovations* (5th ed.). New York: Free Press.

Schein, E. (1992) *Organizational culture and leadership.* San Francisco: Jossey-Bass.

Schein, E. (2010). *Organizational culture and leadership* (4th ed.). San Francisco: Jossey-Bass.

Tiffany, C.R., & Lutjens, L.R.J. (1997). *Planned change theories for nursing: Review, analysis, and implications.* Newbury Park, CA: Sage Publications.

Wheatley, M.J., & Kellner-Rogers, M. (1996). *A simpler way.* San Francisco: Berrett-Koehler Publishers.

8

INTERVENTIONS FOR COMPLEXITY LEADERS

The complexity leader is no longer alone. Others have brought theory to practice, forming a complexity community of support.

■ OBJECTIVES

- Discuss the dynamics and consequences of congruent communication.
- Apply the concepts and process of crucial conversations to health-care leadership practice and interdisciplinary collaboration.
- Explore appreciative inquiry as a method for creating positive change and effective relationships in health care.
- Incorporate the phases of teamwork into improving service and work processes.

INTRODUCTION

Once the complexity leader has a grasp of complex adaptive systems and operates from that perspective, tools are needed. Four are introduced in this chapter. Crucial conversations (Patterson et al., 2002) can help interdisciplinary teams move toward more effective communication, and evidence suggests that better communication and relationships among caregivers of all disciplines affect patient care outcomes positively (Rosenstein and O'Daniel, 2005). Appreciative inquiry (Whitney and Trosten-Bloom, 2003) is another effective approach to communication, relationships, and organizational change that moves the organization from addressing conflicts and problem-based change to one that involves open positive change. The team spirit model (Heermann, 1997) builds teams by incorporating nonlinear concepts with a strong service component. It is an effective vehicle for optimizing relationships and patient care outcomes. Becoming competent in dealing with conflict is addressed in Runde and Flanagan's work on conflict. Basic personal and interpersonal communication concepts are addressed before these four interventions are described.

Common to all of these effective models for bringing groups together in relationship is effective communication.

FOUNDATIONS OF PERSONAL AND INTERPERSONAL COMMUNICATION

All interpersonal communication starts with the personal: what is happening within and how one speaks to and responds to others. Personal communication that is congruent is essential for effective relationships. Congruent communication starts with being aware of what you are experiencing, identifying the feeling associated with the experience, and then honestly articulating those feelings and thoughts in an open way. Automatic defense of your position without first knowing what you believe about a situation or really listening to another blocks the growth toward congruence. Argyris (1993) calls these defensive routines, and they are impediments to honest relationships and block trust.

Joseph Luft and Harry Ingham, two psychologists, created the Johari window (Fig. 8-1) in 1955 as a graphic model of interpersonal awareness (Luft, 1963). The model lends itself to demonstrating how leaders can work toward enhanced congruence through communication.

Figure 8-1 The Johari window. (From Luft, J. [1963]. *Group process: An introduction to group dynamics.* Palo Alto, CA: Mayfield Publishing Company.)

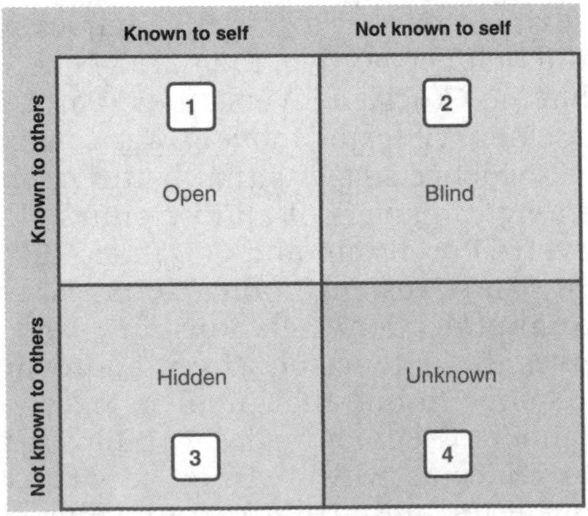

Each quadrant of the window signifies a different combination of the known and unknown.

- Quadrant 1 contains behaviors, qualities, and motivations that are public, known to both self and others. This area signifies shared knowledge.
- Quadrant 2 contains things that others know about you but that you do not know about yourself. It is your blind spot. Everyone has blind spots, or those things others do not tell us. The more open to listening and the less defensive you are, the easier it is for others to give you feedback.
- Quadrant 3 contains things you keep to yourself, the hidden things, the things you do not tell others because of a sense of privacy, decorum, or fear.
- Quadrant 4 is the unknown, with neither party knowing. It is analogous to one's subconscious.

A change in any one of the four quadrants affects the other three. The congruent person has a larger open area in relation to the other three. This means initiating behaviors that decrease the blind spot, being able to receive feedback, and lowering one's façade, as through sharing oneself or self-disclosure. Self-disclosure in relationship to work means being honest with thoughts and opinions when asked for feedback, while maintaining courteous, assertive conversation. It is being able to say the difficult and caring things, which is the hallmark of transforming leaders. Likewise, being able and being known for being willing to receive feedback is incredibly enhancing to one's reputation as an effective leader. It is also the best way to find out what is working and what needs improvement. Listening for feedback is a very effective empowerment device and, for a new leader, establishes the person as someone who can be trusted.

Viewed from a field perspective, self-disclosure and receiving feedback are instances of the leader in a facilitator role. This mutual exchange of disclosure can set the stage for further work in the group.

Congruent Communication in Team Relationships

As previously described, congruence in communication is the process of first experiencing an emotion, identifying it correctly, and communicating that awareness to another honestly. In relationships, there are two ways to be incongruent: not to know one's real feelings and to know but be reluctant to express them (Rogers, 1961).

Being congruent is to be conscious of the emotion that is being experienced. For example, in the first type of incongruence, if a person is angry but not aware of the anger, then another emotion is communicated. This denial is usually because the real emotion is unacceptable to the person for some reason. Most often, when this occurs, others can tell by body language and facial expression what the true feeling is. A person may get quite defensive when the discrepancy is pointed out. This defense mechanism of denial is largely unconscious. In groups, congruent communication is frequently blocked by defensive routines played out from department to department or among team members.

In the other form of incongruence, a person identifies the experienced emotion correctly but is afraid to communicate it. Whereas the first incongruence is denial, the second incongruence is deceit. It may not be intentional deceit, but it is a reflection of fear and mistrust of others. Carl Rogers terms this the existential choice: "Do I dare communicate the full extent of the congruence I feel, or is the risk too great?" (Rogers, p. 345) Incongruence based on denial may be hard to change in a group setting as it is part of an individual's personal makeup, needing individual attention through self-reflection or professional help.

People do have control and choice over expressing their identified true feelings. Creating a field of safety and trust is the challenge for the team leader and the relationship. Setting the tone and creating the field for congruent conversation can be encouraged by understanding and exploring relationship diversities, such as gender, discipline, or mental models. In addition, allowing for various roles and sides of an issue to emerge from within the field enriches the team.

Diversity and Differences

Covey's (1989) habit 5, *Seek first to understand, then to be understood,* is his illustration of congruent conversations. Covey suggests that an agreement among team members to restate another's comments to the other person's satisfaction before replying is an excellent exercise for congruent conversation. When people from different departments or disciplines advocate for their position without listening or seeking feedback, relationships are strained.

In self-organizing systems, there is diversity, and the diversity is for the most part positive. Diverse mental models, power differentials, and identity- or interest-based conflicts call for skill and attention from the complexity leader. Mindell (1995) discusses the reality of power differentials in any group. He calls these issues of rank and privilege. Education, money, and position all influence one's rank and leads to related privilege. Some forms of rank are social status. Other ranks are given by the community or organization such as teacher, parent, or boss. These positions of power are called structural rank. Psychological rank is related to how people feel about themselves, how comfortable and expressive they are with others. Spiritual rank, although more difficult to interpret by others, is related to a person's connection with a higher power or religious sense that sustains the individual in difficult moments. Spiritual rank can be interpreted by others as too much detachment or disinterest in people's everyday concerns.

Sources of conflict can be identity- or interest-based. Identity-based conflicts are those that involve dignity, values, language, family, community, or culture. These sensitive conflicts require empathy and skill to intervene and settle and are more difficult than interest-based conflicts, which are less personal. Interest-based conflicts are more easily handled with the linear, mediator, step-by-step process (Porter-O'-Grady and Malloch, 2007).

In groups we tend to identify ourselves in a certain way, and we hold to that identity and role. Mindell (1995) employs his process work to explain groups. It is difficult to express the other sides of ourselves, to live out those aspects. These less valued (to ourselves) parts of our experience are called the edge, or the border of our personal identity. When we find a situation or an expression of ourselves uncomfortable, we are at the edge. When working with groups, we think in terms of fields. The fields form the patterns, and everything is part of the field. Just as the atmosphere of a meeting can have many different patterns and feelings, and everyone there is part of the field, no one can remain removed from it. As we each express ourselves in a group, we become a channel for the field. When a group has an identity, for example, it believes it always works in harmony, and then when things are not harmonious, the group will disavow that experience because it clashes with the group's perceived identity. But by working things through, going "over their edge," the group can remain whole in the long run. In group life, the parts of the group appear as roles. The field is balanced if all roles in the field are taken up and expressed. This is what happens when a group finds itself without a leader and someone steps up to take on the leadership role. An organization as a whole or a set of groups can only be effective as long as it is successful at working through conflicts and appreciating differences.

Conflict Competence

Runde and Flanagan (2007) offer a model for becoming a conflict-competent leader. Their model exemplifies the personal being and awareness inherent in complexity leadership. They articulate constructive and destructive ways to respond to conflict, and further classify each of these into active or passive behaviors. The active constructive behaviors that lead to a reduction in tension are perspective taking, trying to understand the other's view, creating solutions, not focusing on who is to blame but working with the other toward solutions, and expressing emotions by being open and honest about feelings. The fourth active constructive behavior is reaching out and involves being willing to offer conciliatory gestures in order to open communication. The passive constructive behaviors are less overt, more internal, and more about withholding action. These are reflective thinking, looking at the pros and cons; delay in responding to let emotions cool; and adapting, which involves flexibility, allowing for adjustments, and remaining positive. All of these are facilitated with self-awareness and being open to learning effective communication skills, as well as developing and using personal tools such as centering and self-reflection.

The active destructive behaviors start with winning at all costs, followed by displaying anger, demeaning others, and retaliation. Withholding actions that might help to ease the situation are classified as passive destructive. Avoiding conflict, yielding, hiding emotions, and being self-critical are all aspects of the flight response and interfere with effective leadership.

Runde and Flanagan describe the dynamics of conflict that flow from a precipitating event. One can choose to lean toward constructive behavior, which is more cognitive and task-focused in nature. By focusing on the problem and holding a positive affect, tension can be eased and the conflict lessened while group functioning improves. On the other hand, behaviors that prolong the conflict are destructive and are more personal and emotions-laden. This leads to more tension and less effective group functioning while the conflict grows.

The individual conflict competence model (2010) proposes a positive behavior cycle of cooling down, regulating emotions, and slowing down as needed to dampen emotions. These actions all lead to the goal of engaging constructively with others. Engaging constructively entails reaching out, perspective taking, listening for understanding, sharing thoughts and feelings, and collaborating to create solutions. As a leader works to become self-aware of his or her behaviors and honestly works to attain this level of personal growth and competence in dealing with conflict, strong leadership qualities will emerge and the leader's ability to deal with others will successfully solidify.

CRUCIAL CONVERSATIONS

The authors of *Crucial Conversations* (Patterson et al., 2002) conducted a study entitled *Silence Kills: Seven Crucial Conversations for Healthcare*. This study was conducted in partnership with the American Association of Critical Care Nurses in 2005. Their work and study, *Dialogue Heals* (2006), is taking hold in health-care organizations and proving to be especially helpful for learning communication skills so that a culture of safety and quality can be created. Building on evidence that most medication errors are caused by mistakes in interpersonal communication, they set out to discover the categories of conversations that were perceived to be most difficult for health-care providers in hospitals. These are broken rules, lack of support, mistakes, incompetence, poor teamwork, disrespect, and micromanagement.

An additional finding was that only 1 in 10 health-care professionals actually speaks up in these situations, and the number who will speak up to physicians is even lower. As more studies show the relationship between the quality of communication and the quality of patient care outcomes, developing the skills to tackle the tough conversations is paramount. A conversation is considered crucial when opinions vary, the stakes are high, and emotions are strong. Crucial conversations have all the ingredients of diverse mental models, power and rank differentials, values, and identity issues. When Patterson and colleagues set out to identify those who were successful in their communication, they discovered that the most effective people were the opinion leaders in their respective organizations. These opinion leaders provided a free flow of relevant information. They expressed openness and feelings, articulated theories, and made it safe for others to engage in a pool of shared meaning. They did so by creating the conditions, in themselves and others, to make dialogue the path of least resistance. Looking for ways to keep the conditions of the conversation safe is an important step and requires being aware of one's responses. When people attack, they are typically feeling unsafe. The more one can notice the conditions surrounding the conversation rather than just the content, the more one can help to keep the conversation safe. People often react in two ways when feeling unsafe, with silence or violence, withdrawal or attack. By noticing not just what is being said but also what is happening, dual-processing the situation can help to get a conversation back on track. Part of paying attention to the conditions of the conversation is monitoring one's own behavior. A general description of the dialogue process demonstrates how it is up to each individual to start with a personal commitment to achieve the best possible outcomes for all concerned.

Start with heart. What do you really want? What are your motives? Do you really want mutual purpose and respect? Work on yourself first.

Make it safe. Avoid masking, understating the issue, avoiding, or withdrawing. Do not control, label, or attack. If others feel unsafe, and there is lessening of mutual respect or purpose, step out and try to bring conditions back to safety. Sometimes this requires an apology or explaining what you *do not* want to do but what you *do* hope to accomplish (contrasting); if these fail, try to look for mutual purpose by using the **CRIB** process:

- **C**ommit to seek mutual purpose, by agreeing to agree and stating your intent to stick with the conversation.

- **R**ecognize the purpose behind strategy. Instead of looking at the different strategies for getting what you want, look for the purpose underneath; what is really the purpose for asking for this? There may be a way to get to a new mutual purpose when this is uncovered. For example, most often when there is a difficult conversation between health-care providers, they both really want what is best for the patient but have different ways of going about advocating for it.
- **I**nvent a mutual purpose. If a mutual purpose cannot be discovered, it is possible to invent one, by agreeing on a more encompassing common goal, one that is more meaningful or rewarding to both sides.
- **B**rainstorm new strategies. As safety is restored, conflict can be replaced with collective creative ideas.

Take charge of your emotions. Notice your behavior by retracing your path. Am I in silence or violence? What emotions are influencing me? What story am I telling myself that is creating these emotions? Do I see myself as a victim or helpless in this situation? What role am I playing in this? What do I really want?

STATE *your path.* Speak persuasively with the following:

- **S**hare your facts. Facts are much less controversial than opinions or conclusions.
- **T**ell your story. Once you have laid out the facts, you can draw conclusions, what you believe is happening. Although this is difficult, if you have thought through your approach, and the facts are self-evident, this step is easier to accomplish. Share your point of view, being careful to look out for things becoming unsafe where you might have to back up to assure the other what you are *not* trying to do.
- **A**sk for others paths. Invite others to give their facts and tell their stories.
- **T**alk tentatively. Use phrases such as "I was wondering" or "Perhaps," which combine confidence with some humility. As one increases one's influence, one can also reduce defensiveness in others.
- **E**ncourage testing. Invite opposing views, and really mean it. If people are not responding after encouragement, play the devil's advocate. Disagree with yourself; what if the opposite is true?

Explore others' paths. Use effective, well-tested communication skills, such as asking, actively listening, paraphrasing, and exploring. In crucial conversation terms, these are ask, mirror, paraphrase, and prime.

Move to action. Decide how to decide, and make an actual plan for follow-through to which all agree.

Although this is an overview of how to conduct crucial conversations, complexity leaders can seek more information from the literature and educators to fully engage their organization to improve relationships with the ultimate goal being to improve patient care and staff satisfaction.

APPRECIATIVE INQUIRY

Appreciative inquiry is a method that brings people together to create a climate of interaction where all are heard and honored. Based on social constructionist theory that proposes that people build reality together by language, appreciative inquiry involves the belief that words create worlds in a socially interactive process. Appreciation is the recognition and affirmation of strengths, assets, and potentials. Inquiry is the discovery of what is unknown through exploration of possibilities, being open and willing to learn from one another.

Essential to appreciative inquiry is the belief that people bring unique gifts and skills and, in a social system, unlimited relational capacity. People can create images of the future that will serve to guide their actions and show that attention can be shifted from a focus on problems to a focus on productive future possibilities. A self-organizing complex adaptive system is best suited for employing appreciative inquiry because individual and collective values can be identified, clarified, appreciated, and confirmed. Appreciative inquiry values people as people and not as machines. As they are encouraged to share their successes and hopes, organizational and individual power is released (Whitney and Trosten-Bloom, 2003).

As the system moves from a deficit model to a positive-change model, a positive focus on the potential in the system can be seen. Existing strengths and hopes are shared. The positive core of the organization is identified and amplified. In a paradoxical fashion, as the positive focus occurs, people and the organization are transformed without the specific aim to change anything. In a deficit-based process, the classic problem-based cycle takes place and is often conducted by an outsider. It consists of identification of the problem, selection of the people to solve it, action research, development of best solutions, and then implementation and measurement. In contrast, an appreciative inquiry approach is a positive change process that:

- Chooses affirmative topics
- Involves the whole system
- Discovers a positive core
- Is conducted by members
- Has best practices created by those involved
- Creates a collective approach to a better way

- Forms a design for realizing aspirations
- Sees capacity grow for ongoing positive change

Appreciative inquiry is valuable because it builds relationships in which people are known for more than the roles they play. People are heard, respected, and recognized as contributors. They share their stories and aspirations. They choose what and how to contribute to the whole, based on their passions and interests. The result is that people feel supported, and others are inspired to offer resources and pay attention to everyone's contribution. As people are encouraged to join in affirmative conversation, the tone is set for new ways of looking at the situation to emerge. Once an affirmative topic for appreciative inquiry is chosen, the cycle of Discover, Dream, Design, and Destiny (4D) starts:

- Discover: What works best; purposefully affirmative conversations
- Dream: What might be; challenging the status quo; envisioning ideal, effective processes
- Design: What should be; provocative propositions written in the affirmative
- Destiny: What will be; commitment by all participants, personal and organizational

There are many vehicles for working through the 4D cycle, such as one-on-one interviews, small groups, consortiums, summits, learning teams, and progressive meetings held over time. Schools of nursing and community health-care organizations are challenged with coming together in partnership to meet the needs for clinical venues and for bringing the best-prepared new graduates into the profession. Approaching this challenge from the problem angle of scarce resources and different educational philosophies has not been that successful over time. Coming together in an affirmative, positive manner to discover pockets of best performance and share aspirations beyond old paradigms can lead to new designs for creative programs beyond old structures and commitment to action for real transformation. Creative strategies—such as care units dedicated to patient teaching and statewide curriculums—are being generated across the country as people come together with a focus on the positive rather than on the problems. Reinforcing the important role of appreciative inquiry in the nursing academic community for integrating various interests, Moody and colleagues (2007) reflect, "Therefore, each individual or group acknowledges their positive contributions to self and others, while being encouraged to open up to differing points of view and new assumptions" (p. 321). Eight principles (Table 8–1) reflect the complexity view of people and health-care organizations (Whitney and Trosten-Bloom, 2003). Also see *A Case for Complexity*.

Table 8–1	APPRECIATIVE INQUIRY PRINCIPLES

PRINCIPLE	DISCUSSION
Constructionist	Words create worlds; reality is subjective and socially created through language and conversation
Simultaneity	Inquiry is intervention; asking a question creates change
Poetic	People can choose what they study; organizations are like open books, with endless sources of learning
Anticipatory	Images inspire action; a positive future image can affect present-day action
Positive	Positive questions lead to positive change; so do positive affect and social bonding
Wholeness	Whole stories, whole systems bring out the best for a larger collective capacity
Enactment	Acting "as if"; self-fulfilling; enact the future vision in the present
Free choice	People choose the nature and extent of contribution for empowerment

Adapted from Whitney & Trosten-Bloom, 2003.

A CASE FOR COMPLEXITY

At Maine Medical Center in Portland, Maine, the Registered Nurse (RN) Satisfaction Survey showed staff dissatisfaction with communication, patient flow, and conflict resolution between the post-anesthesia care unit (PACU) and the short-stay unit (SSU).

The nurse director and nurse managers from each unit met with a training and development specialist (TDS) to discuss a plan for building positive relations between the PACU and SSU. Being a Magnet institution, management wanted to empower staff to work together to create a plan. Four staff RNs from each unit volunteered to represent their respective units on an interdepartmental team. The TDS interviewed the eight RNs individually to identify their expectations for interdepartmental teamwork.

The nurse managers took on the shared role of team leader. The TDS acted as the facilitator, and a representative from Human Resources and the eight RNs attended these meetings. The team's first meeting was held in October 2008. Team members quickly identified the current barriers to a collaborative, patient-centered

Continued

A CASE FOR COMPLEXITY—cont'd

work environment and the positive behaviors the team wanted to see in the future. The team began meeting twice a month to address challenges and to plan strategies to achieve and maintain a more collaborative work environment. A team charter was created.

One goal was establishing interdepartmental opportunities for more staff interactions to build relationships, celebrate, and have fun. To accomplish this, the team initiated "random acts of kindness" (bringing cookies to the other department) and planned social gatherings, such as pot luck lunches and cookie swaps. Postcards were created for staff to send to each other following positive interactions. Two collaborative community service projects designed to engage and unite the units were identified. Staff members from each unit participated in two charity walks in the community.

Another goal was to improve staff communication skills to alleviate stress, share information more effectively, and respect professional boundaries. Staff members from each unit identified their need for education to improve their comfort level in addressing and resolving conflict. To this end, a conflict management class was scheduled. Staff members from each unit attended the classes together. A conflict resolution pathway was created to address difficult situations.

Conduct standards were adopted as the norms for both units to establish and promote mutual respect and professionalism in all interactions. Other units were consulted in an effort to gather information as to how conflict was addressed on their units.

Addressing patient flow through the departments was also an important goal for the team. RN staff members from the ambulatory surgery unit and the operating room were asked to join the team for this endeavor. This group was led by a project manager who used a modified value stream mapping process addressing patient flow for late ambulatory unit patients. An algorithm was developed to aid staff in preparing the patient and family as well as standardizing the approach for communication and planning for patient placement/discharge post procedure.

Staff members from both units were kept informed of the team's work through meeting minutes, verbal updates at meetings, and through interactions. A joint meeting for PACU and SSU staff was held a year later to present the team's work in a more formal setting and to allow open discussion among members through panel discussion. Twenty-two staff members attended the meeting. Comments were positive.

In order to assess staff satisfaction in the areas of communication, patient flow, and conflict resolution between the PACU and SSU,

A CASE FOR COMPLEXITY—cont'd

attendees were asked to complete two surveys. One survey inquired about the period before the team completed its goals and implemented strategies for improving the work environment. The second inquired about the period after goals were met and strategies implemented.

The first survey provided a baseline about conflict, accountability, cooperation, and understanding. It reported that 52% of staff members felt conflict was handled in a timely manner, 67% felt they and their peers were held accountable to behave consistently with the organization's values, 74% felt there was good cooperation between the two units, and 61% felt the various staff members made efforts to understand the service needs of the other unit.

The follow-up survey used the same instrument, and the results were favorable. Staff members felt that conflict was handled in a better manner, up to 79%; thus the conflict pathway and classes were a positive. Accountability was somewhat improved, at 68%. Cooperation between the two units rose to 79%. Understanding of service needs increased to 75%.

The survey validated the efforts of the group and also allowed the team to see areas that need to be addressed as next steps. The team continues to meet every month. The staff empowerment approach was successful in building a collaborative patient-centered work environment.

Tara Herman, RN, and Margaret Estee, RN

BUILDING SPIRITED HEALTH-CARE TEAMS

The Team Spirit model (Heermann, 1997) is a nonlinear, field theory–based model that not only deals with team relationships but helps teams to address and improve the quality and service aspects of their work. Teams at their best go far beyond common goals and specific tasks. When discussing team spirit, Heerman states: "In great teams, spirit is manifested in a palpable vitality, purpose, excitement, meaning, and energy. Participation in such teams remains in our consciousness and touches us deeply. It transforms life within and around the team. It is experienced not only as an ephemeral quality of being, but also is an extraordinary record of accomplishment. The spirit in teamwork is ultimately about service and contribution. It is about contribution—generous giving—honoring those we serve with the finest we know how to provide. It is impossible to unravel the interdependency of receiver and giver. Spirit resides in the giving, the receiving, and the ongoing exchange of energy between the team and its customer" (Heermann, 1995, p. 4).

When a team journeys from understanding and acknowledging differences to reflecting on how well members are working together and comes to a shared vision of mutual mission, the team is living the dynamics of a spirited team. The Team Spirit model describes the ingredients and process of becoming a team with spirit. It is a further resource for reflection and growth. Based on organizational development and group process theory, it goes further to include dimensions of spirituality and new science concepts within a framework of accomplishing the actual work of the team.

The traditional, linear organizational development perspective sees team development going through a series of organizational stages in which each stage must be successfully worked through by the team before moving on to later stages. If concerns remain unresolved, for instance, if some level of trust and knowing one another does not occur, the group will remain in the earlier stage and will have difficulty moving on. With team spirit, this is less linear and more holistic.

Scientifically, a team is a rhythmic field with its own set of harmonic qualities, some dissonant, some consonant. Just as in a system, the team evolves. It may go through chaotic, confusing times, which are a part of being a self-organizing system, but it moves toward higher levels of order and harmony. From a spiritual perspective, a team can be seen as an expression of human spirit. In a search for meaning and purpose, people encounter both the awe and wonder of celebrating experiences and encounters with the darker side. Allowing both sides full expression brings the team from dissonance and chaos to a spirited group experience.

In relationships, there is something beyond the performance of tasks to the interactions and mutual growth of teams. Team spirit creates a field in which dynamic relationships flourish. The team spirit spiral (Fig. 8-2) is a model that illustrates the evolving process of building a spirited team. There are five stages or phases: initiating, visioning, claiming, celebrating, and letting go.

Although in some respects this model is developmental when viewed as phases that must be traversed, there is a dynamic quality of the group looping back to relive an earlier stage. And there are times when events and happenings may be a reflection of more than one or all of the phases at the same time because the phases are interdependent. There is a continual ebb and flow, or rhythm, experienced by the team as it builds on its consonances and works through its dissonances (Table 8–2).

The heart of the spiral is service. The consonances of service are contribution, aligned execution, and mutual support. The dissonances

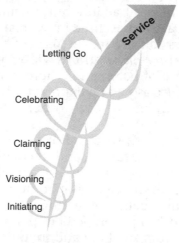

Letting Go

Celebrating

Claiming

Visioning

Initiating

Team Spirit Spiral

Figure 8-2 The team spirit spiral. (From Heermann, B. [1997]. *Building team spirit: Activities for building and inspiring teams.* New York: McGraw-Hill.)

Table 8-2	THE CONSONANCES AND DISSONANCES OF TEAM SPIRIT	
PHASE	**CONSONANCES**	**DISSONANCES**
Initiating	• Belonging • Trust	• Disorientation and alienation • Mistrust
Visioning	• Shared vision and values • Compassion • Presence	• Ambiguous vision and values • Callousness • Aridness
Claiming	• Goal/role alignment • Organizational support • Competence	• Non-alignment • Non-support • Deficiencies in work competencies and outcomes
Celebrating	• Appreciation • Energy • Wonder	• Non-appreciation • Burnout • Disenchantment
Letting go	• Disclosure • Constructive feedback • Completion	• Withheld communication • Criticism • Incompletion

Adapted from Heermann, 1997.

are depletion, uncoordinated action, and unsupportiveness. All aspects of the team field are represented in the team spirit spiral. Learning about each others' differences is part of the initiating phase. Sharing and appreciating each other's viewpoint and orientation builds trust and a sense of belonging. There may certainly be some letting go at this juncture as people express their concerns and move toward more understanding of each other, developing congruent communication.

As the group evaluates its process, discoveries of success and good teamwork will invite celebration and recognition of the team's accomplishments. Self-reflection can also entail some letting go as people express and move through disappointments and frustrations. As it is for many, this new behavior, letting go, requires a skilled, supportive facilitator who has developed enough detachment to allow these roles to emerge from the field and then help the group resolve the issues. The very act of allowing the various roles to emerge will result in a good amount of dissipation of strong feelings.

Visioning is part of mutual mission work. Shared vision is more easily accomplished when differences have been aired, and the group is modeling integration through joint self-reflection. In the claiming phase, doing the work cycles through all others once some basic initiating takes place. If claiming is attempted before some trust and belonging are established and reflection occurs, the work can be stalled or not completed very well. The up-front relationship work will pay off in tasks and projects moving along more smoothly and with fewer personal issues intervening.

The team spirit spiral is an effective evaluation method to use when assessing how well a team is doing. If all five aspects can be demonstrated by a team (and facilitated by the leader) high performance will be evident. If there are problems in the team, determining which phases have not been given sufficient attention is important. A leader/facilitator can employ team-building exercises to reinforce a phase of the spiral. Acting to rectify that lapse can re-energize the team. For example, a team that seems demoralized and discouraged after putting in a great effort that produced good results may have not been encouraged by a leader or allowed itself to recognize its accomplishment through celebration activities. Creating a field where each pulls the others up to a common high standard is enhanced by recognition and celebration.

Roles in the team fields are classified as archetypes in the team spirit model (Table 8–3). An archetype is an essential pattern, invisible field, or prototype that informs behavior, values, actions, and reactions. The archetypes correspond to the phases in the spiral and describe the role a team member plays in regard to the work of the team. When each member fills out the self-assessment to determine his/her archetype

Table 8–3	ARCHETYPES IN THE TEAM SPIRIT MODEL	
ARCHETYPE	PHASE OF SPIRAL	DESCRIPTION
Sower	Initiating	Cultivates relationships
Prophet	Visioning	Reveals possibilities
Protector	Claiming	Ensures results
Elder	Celebrating	Sees good in others
Alchemist	Letting go	Transforms difficulties
Servant	Service	Generously gives

Adapted from Heermann, 1997.

and then shares it with the team, the process can be a powerful team builder. Recognizing and appreciating the contributions of each team member can infuse the team with new spirit.

The team field is about relationships. Relationships within the field can best be explored when individual members are involved in self-development as well. Coming with an ear to listen and willing to identify and then suspend assumptions, each person must commit to discussion and dialogue.

Individuals who are in honest, constructive relationship with others will together create a team with spirit far greater than could be accomplished alone. Reflection on the process of these relationships and how they work together will build health-care teams with greater service and spirit. This can be seen as everyone cares for patients and for each other. As each person learns about and experiences effective team relationships, the knowledge and skill will be transferred to any group or team in the system. There will be an exponential quality to the learning and relating. As soon as it is discovered, any pair or group of people in the health-care system, coming from the same fundamental training and support, will act in coordinated, congruent ways.

Tallia and colleagues (2006) studied medical family practices within a complexity science framework. They searched for the relationship between effective relationships of the providers (interdisciplinary team) and positive patient outcomes. They worked with teams in practices to teach and support effective communication and positive relationships. Their findings have shown that functional work relationships do contribute to successful practices. Furthermore, with considerable research in more than 160 medical practices, they have determined seven interdependent characteristics of successful working relationships. These are trust, diversity, mindfulness, interrelatedness, respect, varied interaction, and effective communication. These represent qualities of an effective complex adaptive system.

- *Trust:* Being open to each other's feedback, allowing people to do their jobs without too much oversight
- *Diversity:* Encouraging diversity in opinions and accepting all kinds of differences in others
- *Mindfulness:* All are open to new ideas and continuously learning and improving
- *Interrelatedness:* Understanding how each person's work affects others and appreciating each other's contributions
- *Respect:* Being considerate, tactful, and honest, even in challenging situations
- *Varied interaction:* Social and task interactions are encouraged
- *Effective communication:* Rich (face-to-face/telephone) and lean (e-mails/memos) communication techniques are used appropriately

SUMMARY

The complexity leader is no longer alone in trying to employ complexity concepts from a theoretical perspective. Unit Two draws on a body of successful research and actual tools and interventions from which to learn. There is no reason for leaders to feel alone in bringing complexity ideas to their health-care organizations. With knowledge about communication and conflict in groups and interventions like crucial conversations, appreciative inquiry, and team spirit, there are choices of substance that uphold complexity values. A complexity management team can choose a model or intervention that fits with its culture that will help its relationships to thrive and form the basis for all of its accomplishments.

Creating a climate that is positive, even joyful, with respect, interdependency, service, learning, and growth is the key to success (Huber et al., 2003). Unit Three focuses on the third component of the complexity leadership model: personal being and awareness. Personal qualities of presence, emotional intelligence, self-awareness, congruence, and life balance are discussed. There are opportunities to assess your own congruence, life balance, and complexity leadership profile.

QUESTIONS FOR SELF-REFLECTION

1. Can you recall a time when in a discussion with others on the team you had an opinion but withheld it (incongruence or deceit) because of anxiety or not having the skill to state your opinion? Describe the situation.
2. When you are in a difficult conversation, do you fall back on silence or violence to feel safe, or are you able to be the one who creates safety for others?

Self-Reflection: What Have I Learned?

_____

_____

_____

_____

_____

8–1   CRITICAL THINKING CASE FOR COMPLEXITY ▬▬▬▬

R.S. is the nurse manager of a large (40-bed) medical-surgical unit at Big Metropolitan Hospital (BMH). She was hired 2 years ago by BMH's chief patient care officer (CPCO). Before her current employment, R.S. was an assistant nurse manager at a hospital that had received many accolades for its stellar nursing care and patient safety record. BMH's hiring process was thorough and included interviews with high-level management personnel as well as with unit staff. The hiring committee was similarly democratically composed and inclusive.

In choosing R.S., the CPCO passed over an internal candidate, M.B., who was the unit's acting nurse manager. M.B, having been a nurse on the unit for over 25 years, is very popular with the unit staff. M.B., along with many of the unit's nurses, received her training at BMH's now-defunct diploma nursing school. Although a very experienced and skilled nurse, M.B. had never pursued education beyond her diploma. In contrast, R.S. recently completed her master's degree. Despite the fact that the CPCO made it clear from the start that the position required advanced nursing education, many of the unit staff viewed the CPCO's hiring decision as arbitrary and discriminatory. Another opinion voiced by staff was that R.S. was an "outsider" and could not understand the needs of the unit.

The CPCO announced her choice and then, having confidence in R.S., turned her attention to other matters. She assumed that R.S. was skilled enough to overcome the staff's resentment.

Shortly after joining the unit, R.S. initiated a new unit nursing model, basing her decision on knowledge gained in graduate school and previous experience. Without much discussion or staff involvement, she hired A.J. as a clinical nurse leader and charged her with improving patient safety and care quality. The position did not carry any line authority.

A.J. began her work on the unit, at first working closely with R.S., to solve some serious unit problems. The staff, although at first outwardly friendly to A.J., gradually began to resist change. Despite dutifully attending required staff education, they refused to alter their practices, some of which were known to be dangerous or negligent.

Despite a lack of staff support, A.J. was able to make some progress, mainly by working with staff from other departments and around unit staff. Patient satisfaction scores rose enough to attract the attention of hospital management. When A.J.'s success was recognized, staff members intensified their campaign against A.J. She became the object of vicious gossip. At A.J.'s first peer review, some staff accused her falsely of falsifying patient satisfaction data in order to show improvement under her leadership.

As conditions on the unit continued to deteriorate, A.J. noticed that R.S. spent more and more of her time either closeted in her office or off the unit. A.J. went to R.S. and asked for her help in managing the staff. R.S. acknowledged the difficulties A.J. faced and sympathized, saying, "Those people will never change." She expressed her hope that "over time" the makeup of the staff would change and "things would improve." She declined to discipline even the worst offenders, citing the long process required to terminate staff and anticipated difficulties in replacing them. R.S. advised A.J. to "figure out" a way to deal with the troublemakers and suggested that A.J. make an effort to be "more friendly" to the staff.

Staff members sensed that R.S. was not inclined to intervene, and they became increasingly defiant. They began to go, individually or in groups, to R.S. to complain about A.J., her ideas, and her actions. Many of these accusations were false and vicious, but R.S. took the easy way out by acting in a conciliatory manner toward the staff and thus not effectively supporting A.J. or the clinical nurse leader role.

Patient care began to suffer, and a crisis soon emerged on the unit. A patient fell and was seriously injured while staff members, including M.B., were gossiping in the hallway about A.J. and R.S. A meeting was held to investigate the incident. The CPCO attended the meeting and expressed her concerns about the incident and about the work atmosphere on the unit. The staff replied by complaining about A.J., whom R.S. again failed to support. The CPCO praised A.J. for her knowledge and skill and her positive impact on patient satisfaction, but she said that A.J. had "poor interpersonal skills." It was suggested that the problem could be solved by A.J. attending some additional training in "working with difficult people."

Claire Lindberg, PhD, RN, FNP, BC

8–2   CRITICAL THINKING QUESTIONS ▰▰▰▰

Using concepts from complexity science, analyze the case study as follows:

1. Describe the situation on the unit, including the origins of the staff's disruptive behavior.
2. Examine the decisions and actions made by the hospital leaders and unit leaders. Discuss failures in leadership and/or in the

system that may have contributed to the disintegration of interpersonal relationships and, subsequently, patient safety and quality of care.

3. Suggest some complexity science–based alternatives or interventions from this chapter to the above decisions and actions, and describe how these alternatives might have led to better outcomes.

REFERENCES

Argyris, C. (). 1993 *Knowledge for action*. San Francisco: Jossey-Bass.

Covey, S.R. (1989). *The 7 habits of highly effective people*. New York: Simon and Schuster.

Heermann, B. (1997). *Building team spirit: Activities for building and inspiring teams*. New York: McGraw-Hill.

Huber, T.P., Godfrey, M.M., Nelson, E.C., et al. (2003). Microsystems in healthcare: Part 8. Developing people and improving work life: What front-line staff told us. *Jt Comm J Qual Safety, 29*(10), 512-522.

Luft, J. (1963/1984). *Group processes: An introduction to group dynamics* (3rd ed.). Palo Alto, CA: Mayfield Publishing Company.

Mindell, A. (1995). *Sitting in the fire: Large group transformation using conflict and diversity*. Portland, OR: Lao Tse Press.

Moody, R.C., Horton-Deutsch, S., & Pesut, D. (2007). Appreciative inquiry for leading in complex systems: Supporting the transformation of academic nursing culture. *J Nurs Educ, 46*(7), 319-324.

Patterson, K., Grenny, J., McMillan, R., et al. (2002). *Crucial conversations: Tools for talking when stakes are high*. New York: McGraw-Hill.

Porter-O' Grady, T., & Malloch, K. (2007) *Quantum leadership* (2nd ed.). Sudbury, MA: Jones & Bartlett Learning.

Rogers, C.R. (1961). *On becoming a person*. Boston: Houghlin Mifflin.

Rosenstein, A.H., & O'Daniel, M. (2005). Disruptive behavior and clinical outcomes: Perceptions of nurses and physicians. *Am J Nurs, 105*(1), 54-64.

Runde, C.E., & Flanagan, T.A. (2007). *Becoming a conflict competent leader*. New York: John Wiley and Sons.

Runde, C.E., & Flanagan, T.A. (2010). *Developing your conflict competence*. San Francisco: Jossey Bass.

Tallia, A.F., Lanham, H.J., McDaniel, R.R., et al. (2006). Seven characteristics of successful work relationships. *Fam Pract Manage, 113*(1), 47-50.

VitalSmarts. *Silence kills: The seven crucial conversations for healthcare*. Retrieved April 18, 2010, from http://www.vitalsmarts.com/dialogueheals.aspx.

Whitney, D., & Trosten-Bloom, A. (2003). *The power of appreciative inquiry: A practical guide to positive change*. San Francisco: Berrett-Koehler Publishers.

Personal Being and Awareness

9

PERSONAL LEADERSHIP SUPPORTING PROFESSIONAL LEADERSHIP

Choosing to become a complexity leader takes more than a little courage. It can feel as if you have cast yourself into a foreign land where others do not think as you do.

■ OBJECTIVES

- Identify the critical role of self-awareness in the complexity leadership model.
- Apply the characteristics of emotional intelligence to effective leadership.
- Integrate the practice of presence into personal being and awareness.
- Identify the leadership and personal behaviors that correlate with characteristics of a complex adaptive system.

INTRODUCTION

The Complexity Leadership Model is unique in that personal leadership is an integral component, in contrast to other leadership models that focus to a large extent on leadership styles or organizational dynamics. Personal being and awareness are essential to complexity leadership. To just know how a complex system works and to enact leadership behavior using that knowledge without also attending to one's personal well-being is very difficult. Judi Neal (2006) calls those leaders *edgewalkers,* those who often find themselves working between two worlds. The chapters in Unit One provided the theoretical background about complexity science to help you think about organizations as complex adaptive systems. The chapters in Unit Two discussed leadership models, styles, and behaviors from an historical perspective and presented contemporary models that are representative of complexity. Here, in Unit Three, chapters discuss the personal being and awareness needed to support and sustain you on your journey to complexity leadership. Once you understand complexity concepts, view your organization as a complex adaptive system, and lead from that complexity perspective, the next step is to employ personal being and awareness to enhance and support your leadership and yourself personally in life as well as work. This is illustrated in Table 9–1. If the characteristics of a complex adaptive system include certain elements, then leadership requires certain behaviors, and the question to ask is, "What personal being and awareness qualities are needed to be a fully effective complexity leader?"

This chapter makes the case for personal being and awareness and discusses the value of self-awareness in effective leadership. The qualities of being, presence, detachment, and letting go are introduced as

Table 9–1   IF...THEN...WHAT

IF CHARACTERISTICS OF COMPLEX ADAPTIVE SYSTEMS INCLUDE:	THEN THE LEADERSHIP BEHAVIOR WILL	WHAT PERSONAL BEING AND AWARENESS QUALITIES ARE NEEDED?
Diverse independent agents interact and adapt to change locally	Invite solutions and ideas from the edge/ from the point of service, not top down	Presence Detachment Letting go
New behaviors, ideas, patterns, and structure emerge from relationships	Create the environment for people to connect and relationships to flourish	Presence Detachment Letting go
Results are often nonlinear, unpredictable, and surprising	Be open to and reward the unexpected positives and refrain from blaming when events are not favorable	Presence Detachment Letting go
Self-organization occurs with distributed leadership and simple rules	Provide only the rules that are needed	Presence Detachment Letting go

elements characteristic of edgewalkers, emotional intelligence, and complexity leaders. Chapter 10 contains the wheel of life, a self-reflective device that brings together concepts and practices of personal being and awareness to help better balance your life. Chapter 11 is devoted to additional self-reflective work to enhance self-care and personal effectiveness. Chapter 12 provides the opportunity to assess your complexity leadership knowledge with summaries and self assessments.

SELF-AWARENESS

The popular television series *The Office* portrays a boss with little awareness of his own actions or of the effect he has on others. Although providing an exaggerated portrayal, this program highlights how essential self-awareness is to effective leadership. Self-reflection is the tool most useful in developing self-awareness. One skill is to develop the ability to meta-communicate with yourself, to think about how you are thinking and observe how you are acting in a given situation. Being able to tune into your mind, bodily sensations, and emotions is a hallmark of self-awareness (Goleman, 1995). Self-awareness is a key component in Goleman's *Emotional Intelligence* (1995) and in Neal's *Edgewalkers* (2006). Both will be described as exemplifying complexity leadership qualities.

Following are two scenarios (see *A Case With Two Outcomes*), one where the leader has not incorporated personal being and awareness into his daily living leadership and the same situation if he were a fully practicing complexity leader.

People with emotional awareness recognize their emotions and how the expression of these emotions affects others. They understand why they are feeling these emotions and see the link between them and what they think, do, and say. They are guided by their values and goals and understand how their feelings affect their performance (Goleman, 1995). Although self-awareness is a commonality between edgewalkers and those with emotional intelligence, there are traits particular to each. Both will be described in more depth as well as their relationship to complexity leadership.

Edgewalkers

Neal (2006) describes an edgewalker as often in the position of being between two worlds with differing views and perspectives about organizational leadership. Edgewalkers are people and organizations that take risks, build bridges, and break new ground. Edgewalkers have a quality of being that sets them apart, especially a heightened self-awareness, of being aware of thoughts, values, and behaviors. Edgewalkers possess other qualities of being that reflect

A CASE WITH TWO OUTCOMES

Scenario 1

Jerry was the director of two departments. He was preparing to attend a meeting where the departments had a disagreement about a course of action. Both sides had asked him to attend. They viewed him as a very good facilitator who walked the talk of distributed leadership. He believed that an important leadership role for him was to create a safe place for people to discuss their diverse opinions openly and that a better solution would be found with his support and their willingness to engage.

Jerry felt a bit stressed going into the meeting, but he brushed it off. "I need another cup of coffee," he thought. As the meeting progressed, Jerry felt increasingly uneasy, and this distracted him from being present to the group. Each side retreated to its own positions, the issue became more muddled, and finally, with time up, they adjourned after scheduling another meeting for the following week. All left the room wondering how things had fallen apart and felt a bit dejected. Jerry didn't feel like a complexity leader at all.

Scenario 2

As Jerry prepared for his meeting, he noticed he was unusually anxious about it. He thought, "Hmm. This isn't the type of situation that I normally get anxious about. I wonder why I feel this way." He paused, became centered for a moment and, with this time and space to introspect, realized that he very decidedly favored one department over the other in this issue. As soon as he had that insight, he could put it all back into perspective and remind himself of the neutral helpful role he needed to play. Jerry took a minute to breathe and center himself, and he reframed his thinking to one of reaffirmation of his leadership role. In the meeting, with his open supportive inquiring stance, he was able to really be present. Both sides felt safe to explore the issue at hand, and they even asked Jerry's opinion, which he was able to voice without forcing his ideas. There was a nice balance of advocacy and inquiry. People became animated and excited about the possibilities as they developed a plan of action built on the best ideas from all perspectives. They left the meeting feeling good about all they had accomplished.

complexity leadership. They are passionate and lead with integrity, vision, and playfulness. They have an intense focus on passion and purpose in life and work. Neal found through interviews that edge-walkers often have had difficult childhoods or some transforming life event. This is similar to Collins's (2001) description of Level 5 leaders (see Chapter 6). Some revelation or deep personal work has planted that seed that brings these leaders to another level of being. Passionate leaders can motivate others to engage in meaningful activities when they feel that they are involved in and connected to an idea or cause greater than themselves.

Integrity involves being in alignment with one's core values and then acting in concert with those values; being committed to keeping one's word. Carl Rogers (1961) termed this alignment of thoughts, feelings, and behaviors as *congruence*. Self-awareness through self-reflection is paramount to first getting in touch with one's own core values before one can act with integrity.

The vision that edgewalkers have goes beyond setting goals and strategic planning. They see possibilities, tapping into spiritual sources for inspiration. Edgewalkers and complexity leaders spend time in contemplation and personal self-reflection, which helps them remain present and centered while working with others. They are able to see the patterns and connections and ideas that are emerging, even when events seem chaotic.

Finally, edgewalkers are open to surprise, not knowing all the answers and greeting these circumstances with good humor and flexibility. They are playful, keeping things in perspective. There is a celebratory aspect to their being, similar to the archetypal elder who sets a tone for celebration in the team-spirit model of team building (see Chapter 8). An interesting paradox is in play with edgewalkers and complexity leaders who attend to personal being and awareness. They have a passion for the work and a sense of detachment for the outcome at the same time. Detachment involves suspension of judgment, not labeling things good or bad, but just seeing them as they are. Passion, excitement, and strong beliefs are the greatest motivations for living fully. If you can keep the passion without taking an emotional nosedive each time there is a disappointment, change in plans, or less than desirable outcome, then you are generating the quality of detachment. The quality of detachment is addressed in Chapter 10.

Emotional Intelligence

In *Working with Emotional Intelligence,* Goleman (1998) goes beyond discussing the origins and traits of emotional intelligence to describing the essential emotional and social competencies in his emotional competencies framework. Table 9–2 presents the key points of the framework.

In Goleman's original inquiry into what held less effective leaders back, two themes emerged: rigidity and poor relationships. These unsuccessful leaders could not adapt to changes in organizational culture, and they did not listen to others or accept feedback. Their

Table 9–2	EMOTIONAL COMPETENCE FRAMEWORK
PERSONAL COMPETENCE	
How one manages oneself	*Self-awareness:* Knowing one's internal states, preferences, resources, and intuitions *Self-regulation:* Managing one's internal states, impulses, and resources *Motivation:* Emotional tendencies that guide or facilitate reaching goals
SOCIAL COMPETENCE	
How one handles relationships	*Empathy:* Awareness of others' feelings, needs, and concerns *Social Skills:* Adeptness at inducing desirable responses in others

From Goleman, 1998.

propensity to be critical, insulting, and demanding toward others led to alienation. They lacked self-control, were moody, and did not handle pressure very well. They blamed others and were defensive. Highly ambitious, they would readily push ahead at the expense of others. These failing leaders, lacking empathy and sensitivity to others, could be arrogant and, even if appearing caring, it was only to be manipulative. All of these shortcomings blocked their ability to build networks or cooperative relationships and to appreciate and encourage diversity in mental models and discipline perspectives. This array of ineffective traits clearly is the antithesis of not only emotional intelligence but of the complexity leader.

With attention to personal being and awareness, complexity leaders can achieve emotional and social intelligence. These effective leaders are able to achieve self-control, allowing them to remain calm and confident under stress and chaotic circumstances. They admit their mistakes and, like Collins's Level 5 leaders, they do not seek to assign blame but address what part they may have played. They are tactful, empathic, and considerate with people at all levels of the organization. Being able to relate and connect to people at all levels of an organization and to create structured empowerment for nurses at all levels are the predominant abilities seen in chief nurse officers in Magnet hospitals (ANCC, 2008). Leaders with emotional and social competence honor diversity and seek to connect and network to form rich relationships in all manner of patterns and in many different circumstances.

Goleman determined there are social skills of an interpersonal nature to enable leaders to be effective, including: the ability to initiate and coordinate the efforts of a network of people, to organize, to mediate disputes to help with group conflicts, to connect and respond to others' feelings and concerns, and, in general, to develop the art of the relationship.

NOBLE PURPOSE

Noble Purpose (Heermann, 2004) is a program that employs self-reflection and self-awareness to help people uncover their work/life purpose. It is based on the team-spirit model described in Chapter 8, using the phases of team development—initiating, visioning, claiming, celebrating, and letting go—but applied to personal development and self-discovery. A leader seeking a self-reflective process may find this program valuable. The basic elements are presented as a possible vehicle for taking a self-reflective journey as it incorporates essentials of personal being and awareness: presence, detachment, and letting go.

A starting premise of Noble Purpose is one based on psychological theory. Through self-awareness, a person can find and tread the path to the essential self. The essential self has often been blocked by some dissonance that developed in the past from difficult experiences. A person then protects oneself with an outer shell—in Noble Purpose, the bounded self. As people engage in the Noble Purpose process, they regenerate passion and purpose to live and work meaningfully and with an aim of being of service to others and to causes greater than themselves. The Noble Purpose phases are:

- *Initiating*—Choosing the path of belonging and trust, knowing your universe is perfectly unfolding
- *Visioning*—Discovering your passion and purpose, visualizing it in the world
- *Claiming*—Being accountable and responsible for manifesting your vision
- *Celebrating*—Experiencing the joy of knowing your life makes a difference
- *Letting go*—Releasing fear and need for power, control, and approval

With initiating, one delves deeply for inner knowledge, to be present and to trust oneself on examining one's dissonances. The aim of the work in this phase is to release evaluation and judgment of self, others, and circumstances. It is important to acknowledge gifts and resources and to trust that life and work are perfect as they are.

Visioning, putting energy and passion into finding one's purpose, is difficult before the initiating process is completed. Resolving tendencies to be self-critical must come first. Trying to be energized and inspired while at the same time being self-critical puts one in a state of cognitive dissonance, unable to move forward and having diminished energy. Once one is mostly free of this, then one can become conscious of one's sources of energy and interests. One is open to looking for inspiration and visualizing the best future.

The work of claiming involves the actual doing of one's chosen work, from planning through execution. There is a caution here, however. Three threats to claiming may exist: too much need for power and control, being fixated on results, and needing to look good. These clearly will get in the way of one's journey to complexity leadership. They are traits that are in opposition to such complexity thinking as distributed leadership, self-organization, uncertainty, and forming rich relationships.

Celebrating is the next phase. Individual and collective energy are enhanced when people celebrate, appreciate, value, and acknowledge the work they do. The appreciative inquiry process is an example of a fulfilling celebration process.

There are two aspects to letting go. The first is relationship-based: effective communication that leads to resolving difficulties and painful situations with others. The second is the inner work of releasing childhood wounding, the fundamental dissonance that can be uncovered with deep personal self-reflection and a commitment to the Noble Purpose process. So much of letting go is noticing—being self-aware of responses and reactions. Are there times when you do not engage because of fear of failure or disapproval? Do you use power, control, or manipulation to achieve results? Are you able to be congruent in your communication, both disclosing feelings and giving constructive feedback?

Noble Purpose is a form of inner work. Inner work prepares leaders to enter into groups and relationships from a more centered perspective, to be calm, open, and present even when there is conflict and chaos. Often, inner work—for instance, a personal decision to change behavior toward another—may yield results even before there is an outward change in behavior, so powerful is the effect of personal being and awareness on relationships with others.

PRESENCE

Eckhart Tolle asks, in *The Power of Now* (1999), if one treats any given moment as if it were an obstacle to overcome, is there a future moment to get to that is more important? A vital key to personal being and awareness and ultimate effectiveness as a complexity leader is the ability to be present, to practice presence, and to be present to each moment, situation, and person. The presence required for true nurse caring is the same that is needed for complexity leadership. McCrae (2001) relates four levels of nurse presence:

1. Physically present—no interaction; self-absorbed
2. Partially present—notices and greets but then goes about tasks
3. Full presence—attentive, listening, focused on the here and now
4. Transcendent presence—peaceful, comforting, transforming, and harmonious connection/energy beyond the interaction of the two

Level 3 should be the operating level for complexity leaders at all times. Level 4 may arise on occasion and should be encouraged when it occurs. Transcendent presence happens usually when two or more people are fully present and engaged with passion, excitement, or flow. It is that unique coming together of people who move a team or an organization to extraordinary heights. A leader's ability to maintain Level 3 in everyday practice serves as an attractor for others to develop the trust to expect that level of interaction consistently.

Presence and self-awareness are partners. Self-awareness can only be achieved by being in the present moment, by being the watcher of your mind, reactions, thoughts, and emotions (Tolle, 1999). This is mindfulness, nonjudgmental awareness of the present moment. Time spent in the past, either lamenting failures or reliving successes, or time and attention thrust into the future leads away from being fully in the moment. Tolle calls this *psychological time*. It is easy to build up psychological time by bringing old hurts and memories from the past and projecting them into the future. Learning from the past is valuable, but then apply the lesson in the present for new behavior. Similarly, one cannot be fully present either if one lives ahead of oneself into the future, whether by worrying or daydreaming at the expense of present activity. Tolle observes, "The moment you realize you are not present, you are present" (p. 45). There is actual clock time, which helps with everyday activities, such as setting and achieving goals, but Tolle cautions return to present awareness as soon and as often as possible. One's goals are more easily accomplished when one loses a sense of time and becomes one with the activity of the moment, what Csikszentmihalyi (1990) calls being *in the flow*. Another way to look at the concept of time is to move from considering time as an amount to spend on getting tasks done to considering it as a space that holds current experience.

Senge and colleagues (2004), in *Presence: Human Purpose and the Field of the Future*, first identified presence as self-awareness of the moment but then moved to discovering that presence is also deep listening, a willingness to suspend judgment, and letting go of old identities. From deep understanding of the present, one can create the future. This can be a personal presencing, a deep inner knowing, or a collective effort, being present to each other and the moment where new ideas emerge.

Being present in the moment has the added bonus of enhancing time management. As one remains present to the person or activity, one accomplishes more in a shorter time. Being present is a valuable ally in setting and attaining goals. To do this, set goals in the present. This means not setting a goal to accomplish in the future—"Tomorrow, I will..."—because the subconscious accepts that as always in the future, never to be done. Instead, develop a new approach to *now*. For example, for a goal of healthy eating, do not say, "I am going to start eating more vegetables"; rather, "I am a person who eats several helpings of vegetables a day." In the interpersonal realm, this can be very effective in everyday leadership. "I am a person who listens fully, is open to new ideas, is not overly attached to outcomes, and invites many diverse ideas." Tolle (1999) reflects that by becoming friends with the present moment, one feels at home no matter where one is. This feeling "at home" and "at ease" in any situation is the ultimate quality for effective complexity leadership as well as personal contentment and fulfillment. This chapter's *Case for Complexity* describes an organizational consultant who, through self-awareness and being a watcher of her mind, achieved a successful interaction with a client.

A CASE FOR COMPLEXITY

Influencing the Environment: Using Self-Awareness to Turn Adversaries Into Partners

I entered the meeting with some trepidation. The physician was a member of a multidisciplinary team and, by all accounts, was intelligent and highly skilled. He was also reputedly demanding and quick to find fault. My assignment was to help the team resolve an internal conflict that had polarized its members and resulted in stilted communication, lack of trust, and concern about patient care. I was hired by management, which included the physician. The purpose of this meeting was to present the results of a comprehensive instrument and, specifically, how his ratings of himself compared with those of peers and employees.

There was a wide gap in perceptions. The physician saw himself as flexible, constructive, and an able communicator. Peers and employees feared his judgment and disliked his aloofness and rigidity.

A CASE FOR COMPLEXITY—cont'd

I arrived early and was seated in the waiting room. About 20 minutes after the scheduled appointment time, a staff person said the physician would be with me shortly. Fifteen minutes later, I was directed to his office. The other interviews had started on time, with the interviewee escorting me to his or her office. I found my way to a long hall at the end of which stood the client. As I approached, I said hello and greeted him by name. He said nothing. I followed him into his small office. There was one desk and chair–his–and a couch perpendicular to the desk and far enough away to make a presentation difficult. As he sat down, he directed his body toward the desk and away from me. I asked if we could sit so that he could see the materials more easily. He indicated nonverbally that he was fine. These seemingly obvious breeches of professional courtesy seemed astounding, yet there I was, expected to make a presentation to someone barely looking at me and who seemed not remotely interested in research he had hired me to do. By his conscious or unconscious design, he was letting me know that he held all the power, that my report and I were meaningless intrusions on his busy day, and that the sooner this was over the sooner he could get back to important items on his agenda.

I realized if I was going to do the job for which I was hired, I needed to take charge of the environment in a more purposeful way. I thought about the martial art I practice and teach–Aikido–in which the goal is to align with and redirect the attacker's energy. By aligning, instead of resisting, one regains power and can control the attack without harming the attacker.

I started to align by stating my interpretation of the desired outcomes for the intervention and asked if he saw things in a similar way. (Yes, he did. Excellent.) I explained that, for me, it was important that he be able to see the data in the report and follow along as I described the process. I opened the door to his office, found a chair in the hall, and positioned it so that we were now side by side.

Next, I invited his energy with open-ended questions. I wanted to find areas that sparked interest. What did he think was the purpose for our session? What would be his ideal outcome? Which parts of the instrument interested him most?

Gradually, and with subtle choices, I began to reinvent the environment. Regardless of what the physician said, I stayed curious. When he offered verbal or nonverbal resistance, I acknowledged and redirected it toward our stated mutual purpose. Most important, I refused to become an opponent. I continued to configure our relationship as partners who were attempting to solve a problem together,

Continued

A CASE FOR COMPLEXITY—cont'd

and little by little he joined me in that endeavor. He saw that I was not there to expose or criticize but to support. It was a valuable learning experience in the malleable nature of relationship and reinforced my personal belief that when people change, everything changes. We create our environment moment to moment. When we know this to be true, we can become more intentional about the process.

Judy Ringer
*Author, *Unlikely Teachers: Finding the Hidden Gifts in Daily Conflict*

SUMMARY

In describing personal being and awareness, who one is determines how one leads. Inner work makes all the difference. Chapter 10 provides an opportunity for inner work and discovery about balance in life. This chapter ends with a poem written by a graduate nursing student in a course about leadership in complex systems and used with her permission.

QUESTIONS FOR SELF-REFLECTION

1. Can I be patient when a situation looks disorganized and uncertain?
2. Can I let go and be present while others bring out their ideas?
3. What part might I have played in a difficult situation?

When I Know Who I Am

When I know who I am,
Understand that my decisions do matter
And affect others
Even those that I do not know,

And make a conscious effort to be
In relation with others,
Then I will become the leader

At any level
In which I live
In that moment

—LYNN GEOFFRION

Self-Reflection: What Have I Learned?

_____

_____

_____

_____

_____

9–1 CRITICAL THINKING QUESTION ▰▰▰▰

Review Table 9–1. Select one of the characteristics and corresponding leadership behaviors. Based on your selection, describe a leadership situation in which the leader was either very effective or not effective, depending on the behavior and actions of that leader.

9–2 CRITICAL THINKING CASE
FOR COMPLEXITY ▰▰▰▰

I am a psychiatric nurse practitioner; I was asked to evaluate Mrs. T., a 76-year-old female who was admitted to the emergency department (ED) for a chief complaint of falling and dizziness. The patient was described to me by the ED nurse as "agitated, upset, confused, and disoriented to person, place, and date." The ED physicians had cleared the patient medically, so she was turned over to me to see if I could assess her for dementia, underlying delirium, or superimposed depression on delirium and dementia, all of which were possible. I spoke to the ED physician and nurse, both of whom thought the patient had a mental health issue, but I did not assume that. I centered myself and looked afresh at the patient and her circumstances. I reviewed the laboratory test results, which showed she had a low sodium level. She appeared to be dehydrated, as evidenced by her skin turgor and frequent lip smacking. Her husband said she was drinking a lot of water.

Her head computed tomography scan result was normal, and her urine screen was normal. Her urine toxicology was positive for benzodiazepines, but she was taking Ativan 0.5 mg at bedtime. Her oxygen saturation was 94%, but according to her husband this was normal for her. Her electrocardiogram and chest x-ray were also normal.

After reviewing her medical record, I went in to see Mrs. T. She was accompanied by her husband, who was loving and caring and who had genuine concern for his wife. He said, "This was pretty sudden. She was just diagnosed with early dementia, but the sudden change in her behavior is concerning. I know something else is happening. Can you help us?" I offered assurance that we would do everything possible to try to find the cause of the sudden change in Mrs. T's behavior. I approached Mrs. T, introduced myself and my role as a psychiatric nurse practitioner, and told her I was going to ask her some questions. She knew she was in a hospital, but she did not know she was in the ED, the name of the hospital, or the date. My evaluation consisted of a mental status evaluation and psychiatric history, which indicated that she had long-term anxiety but otherwise no significant mental illness such as depression or hospitalizations for such. A mini-mental examination was administered to assess her cognitive abilities, and on this exam she scored 25 out of 30, which for her age and her early diagnosis of dementia appeared to be a good score.

I asked both Mrs. and Mr. T about her recent use of medications. She said she was having a lot of diarrhea, and she had been taking Imodium daily. Mr. T said that he had witnessed Mrs. T taking several doses of Imodium a day for the last 3 days. In addition, Mrs. T stated she was taking Tylenol PM every night to help her sleep, because the Ativan was no longer effective. As I began to uncover the rationale for the use of Tylenol PM and the frequent use of Imodium, it occurred to me that her symptoms were indicative of anticholinergic syndrome. The classic symptoms of this syndrome are "mad as a hatter, red as a beat, and dry as a bone." She was dehydrated, which was probably from the Imodium, frequent diarrhea with loss of fluid and potassium, and most likely the Tylenol PM, which contains Benadryl and contributes to dehydration. She was very irritable and restless but not out of control. She was slightly warm to the touch; her skin was very dry, and she was extremely thirsty.

Once it was recognized that dehydration was most likely the cause of Mrs. T's rapid change in behavior, the ED physician agreed to admit her for observation and hydration. This clinical situation allowed me to educate the ED staff and Mrs. and Mr. T about the side effects of anticholinergic medications. I was pleased that I had kept present to the patient and her husband, really listened to them, and had not assumed that there was no medical reason for her symptoms. I was gratified that that team respected me; by working together as a team, the ED staff, the patient, her husband, and I were able to find a solution to her behavior. It was essential that we took the time to do these tests and did not pass this patient off as just another confused elderly patient. The ED nurses also completed a thorough assessment, which was instrumental in assisting me in my own assessment. This clinical situation may not have been so easy to diagnose and treat had we not all been a team who came together for the best interest of the patient, and as such we all witnessed a good outcome as a result. We were present for the patient and for each other.

Larry Plant, PMH-NP, BC, DNP(c)

9–3 CRITICAL THINKING QUESTION ◼◼◼◼◼◼

This case illustrates how being present and centered can enhance one's diagnostic capabilities and respect by and for other team members. Describe a time in your practice when there was either a successful or unsuccessful outcome that was related to your being centered and present to the patient and to the team.

REFERENCES

American Nurses Credentialing Center. (2008). *Application manual: Magnet recognition program*. Silver Spring, MD: Author.

Collins, J. (2001). *Good to great*. New York: HarperCollins.

Csikszentmihalyi, M. (1990). *Flow: The psychology of optimal experience*. New York: Harper and Row

Goleman, D. (1995/2006). *Emotional intelligence: Why it can matter more than IQ*. New York: Bantam Books.

Goleman, D. (1998). *Working with emotional intelligence*. New York: Bantam Books.

Heermann, B. (2004). *Noble purpose: Igniting extraordinary passion for life and work*. Fairfax, VA: QSU.

McCrae, J.A. (2001). *Nursing as a spiritual practice: A contemporary application of Florence Nightingale's views*. New York: Springer.

Neal, J. (2006). *Edgewalkers: People and organizations that take risks, build bridges, and break new ground*. Westport CT: Praeger.

Rogers, C.R. (1961/2004). *On becoming a person: A therapist's view of psychotherapy*. London: Constable.

Senge, P.M., Scharmer, C.O., Jaworski, J., et al. (2004). *Presence: Human purpose and the field of the future*. Cambridge, MA: The Society for Organizational Learning.

Tolle, E. (1999). *The power of now: A guide to spiritual enlightenment*. Novato, CA: New World Library.

10

COMPLEXITY LEADERSHIP: PERSONAL AND PROFESSIONAL LIFE BALANCE

The complexity leader is congruent in perspective, action, and being, leading with awareness, intention, and grace.

■ OBJECTIVES

- Apply the concept of congruence to complexity leadership.
- Identify states of congruence for effective personal being and awareness.
- Discover areas of cognitive dissonance in personal and professional life.
- Employ self-reflection to assess personal and professional life balance.

INTRODUCTION

Chapter 9 discussed some key states of personal being and awareness: self-awareness, presence, detachment, and letting go. Chapter 9 also presented emotional intelligence and Noble Purpose as two models that can be employed to develop these states of being. Chapter 10 expands on these states of being through discussions of congruence and cognitive dissonance. You will have opportunities to explore your own areas of congruence and cognitive dissonance.

LEADING THE CONGRUENT LIFE

The core of a balanced personal and professional life is being congruent in two ways. The first is living in congruence with your values and beliefs for the overall scheme of your life. The second is being congruent in your everyday living, your interpersonal congruence. This occurs when your thoughts, feelings, and behavior are consistent and in alignment. Without front or façade, the congruent person can openly express feelings and attitudes as they flow, being truly genuine. Trust is engendered by those who operate from a congruent stance.

Rogers (1961) believed that the greater the congruence of the therapist, the more successful the outcome for the client. There is a parallel here for leader behavior. Clients can better engage with and trust therapists they can rely on to act consistently and honestly and who are comfortable with themselves and others. This is a description of a congruent leader as well. Congruent leaders in their relationships with others can promote growth of individuals and the system within which they practice. Indeed, an entire complex system can move toward greater congruity as those within actualize congruent behavior. In a reciprocal fashion, congruent leaders create an environment, a field where it is safe for people to be themselves, to express true feelings and thoughts about their work. Congruence is not a static state; it is a process of becoming.

In a complex adaptive system, the complexity leader encourages diversity and sets the expectation for open communication. This creates the environment with an ebb and flow of diverse ideas. These ideas may be contrary to the leader's views but, with congruence, challenges can be handled. When leaders are never challenged, this signals an organization that is rigid and uncreative.

Life congruence starts with discovering or uncovering your values and beliefs, then living out those values. For example, living a messy, ineffective, or inauthentic life may not be troubling to you only; it is the way others will perceive you and judge your values. How can people think that your behavior is anything but a reflection of your values and beliefs? How can leaders be perceived as anything other than how they present themselves on a daily basis?

States of Congruence

You may be living in any of the following states in which you:

1. Do not know what you value, and you act in a haphazard and reactive manner
2. Do not know your values and beliefs, and you act based on others' dictates
3. Know your values but for many reasons do not act according to them
4. Know your values and beliefs and act accordingly

The fourth state above—knowing your values and beliefs and acting accordingly—is true congruence. Congruence emerges from a long process of self-reflection and life experiences. People are not always in that full state of congruence. It takes mindful self-awareness. People generally slip and slide back and forth to State 3, knowing what they believe but not acting according to those beliefs. Some reasons may be anxiety, lack of skill in difficult situations, or a life event that makes one less confident. People may revert to State 2, being unsure of what they believe so they then behave based upon what others tell them to do. A move to State 2 may be related to being in a new learning situation and not having the knowledge base or experience to perform at a higher level. There is a developmental challenge to meet in order to move from this to greater congruence. Just as Benner's (1984) model suggests, an expert in one area can revert to a less developed stage—competent or even advanced beginner when put into a new situation. Likewise, from a situational leadership (Beck and Yeager, 2001) perspective, a Level 4 person, while independent, willing, and capable, will need the direction required of a Level 2 when changing to a new position. A review of the four levels of situational leadership follows. Level 1 employees are not able to perform and may or may not be willing to do so. They require the most direction and less relationship support. Level 2 people are usually quite willing to do the work and have some knowledge at this point, so they need both direction and relationship support. There is much less need for direction once a person reaches Level 3, but relationship support is still important. Level 4 people are very independent and very skilled in their performance; thus, they can operate with very little relationship support or direction. A Level 2 person requires both attention to relationship and the direction needed for learning the new task and knowledge. A person in State 1 congruence is in need of much nurturing and developmental help, often of a professional nature. The exception to that is the rare instance when a person may be going through some very unusual spiritual or life crisis and for a period is unable to cope at a higher level.

The developmental progression then for a new leader or one who is moving from linear to complexity leadership involves some form of the following steps. First, start with emulating another's leadership style, without having a firm base of knowledge (State 2). This can produce cognitive dissonance because there are no firm, clear values and beliefs to match or support the behaviors. There can be a sense of unease, as a person tries to act on others' beliefs. Then as one seeks knowledge upon which to build behavior, there is usually a journey through State 3, knowing what one believes and values, but not always acting accordingly. Cognitive dissonance is present here, with a contradiction between beliefs and actions. Cognitive dissonance is described in more detail in the following section. Personal growth is required to develop the skills and self-awareness to become congruent at State 4, to be one's fully authentic self. It takes courage to be that authentic self. When you are certain about what you value and the direction for your life, you can move forth to express yourself congruently. Figure 10-1 demonstrates the four states of congruence and the developmental movement from States 1 to 4.

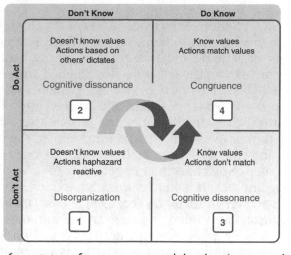

Figure 10-1 The four states of congruence and the developmental movement from States 1 to 4.

COGNITIVE DISSONANCE

Cognitive dissonance is the result of a contradiction or an inconsistency between attitudes, beliefs, and values, and how one behaves (Festinger, 1957). The dissonance is the most evident when a person must choose between two beliefs or actions. This is certainly so with a leader who has come to believe that leading an organization from a complexity perspective is most effective but feels caught in a linear setting. The leader who is in congruent State 3—knowing the values but not acting on them—is also experiencing this cognitive dissonance by having a complexity perspective but not having the skills and competencies to act on that knowledge. The real difficulty with being in a state of cognitive dissonance is the stress and strain emotionally and physically that it creates. It is a significant energy drain and can lead to emotional distress, burnout, and even physical discomfort and illness. Resolution of cognitive dissonance becomes an imperative.

There are two ways to resolve cognitive dissonance: change the thinking, or change the situation. This involves changing the thinking by either rationalizing that the belief or value is not that important or by accepting and tolerating the situation. For example a college student dislikes a part-time job working in a bar because he does not believe in drinking, but it is the only job he could find. He could resolve his cognitive dissonance by either changing his thinking by rationalizing, "After all, I don't drink, so I am okay" or, by refuting the situation, "This is the only job I could find; I need the money, and it is only for one semester." A third way is to change the situation by quitting.

Consider a situation in which a leader is squarely in State 3 congruence. She has been exposed to complexity leaders, attended conferences, and now embraces the complexity perspective. However, she is held back from fully acting as a complexity leader by a combination of lack of skills and a tendency toward wanting control and quick answers. She is clearly missing the personal being and awareness element of complexity leadership. If she embarks on the self-reflection needed and sets out to learn the essential self-reflective practices and interpersonal skills, she will become that complexity leader in action. She is then congruent in perspective, action, and being. In this case, she has neither diminished the importance of the complexity perspective nor refuted the need to change her behavior. Instead, she has actually changed from cognitive dissonance to congruence by changing her behavior to be in alignment with her knowledge and beliefs. Often, choosing to change the situation can be a very dramatic and difficult choice, as in *A Case for Complexity*.

There are reasons for underlying cognitive dissonance. For example, when there is a large gap between the time you spend on an area of your life and your amount of satisfaction, that is a form of cognitive dissonance. You can discover what your true values are by reflecting on this cognitive dissonance. You may be working very long hours and spending little time with your family or on other fulfilling activities. If your satisfaction level is low about this, what does it mean? It may mean that you really do value work above other areas of your life, but then

A CASE FOR COMPLEXITY

René, a seasoned senior nursing leader with well-developed complexity leadership knowledge, skills, and personal being and awareness, finds herself in an organization where the senior leadership and board are still operating in a very linear mode. She is feeling increasingly frustrated with this situation. Her complexity view is not shared by many others, except the small group in her department. In fact, this is what initially drew her to the position.

René has two choices. She can settle, "It's okay, I need this job. I was unrealistic to think things were different here, and besides I have my close associates to gripe with." Alternatively, she can view the situation for what it is, but also see the possibilities, find reason to refute her thinking about the organization, and use her leadership skills to work with like-minded others to move the organization toward complexity.

She understands that small actions at a local level can have large effects. Her personal being and awareness plus rich relationships can sustain her through the process as she reduces her cognitive dissonance in the process. Of course, she can use the third option to reduce her cognitive dissonance—resign the position and find another position in another organization. This third solution sometimes is the only way out of the problem, but for some this becomes a habit, never facing and working through a cognitive dissonance.

to be really congruent, the amount of work and satisfaction would need to be more closely correlated. Perhaps you are living according to others' expectations of what is "good living," and you are not sure about your own values and identity. Uncovering your true values relating to work and the rest of your life sets you back on the path to congruence.

First and essential to a balanced personal and professional life are your values. This entails discovering or uncovering what your true values for living are, then living in congruence with those values. When there is a discrepancy between what you believe to be "rightful" living and the manner in which you do live day to day, you are living in conflict, consciously or unconsciously. This is a form of cognitive dissonance. It drains your energy and keeps you stressed and reactive. There is a clarity and calmness whenever you act according to your beliefs because neither excuses nor defenses are needed.

One way a person can slip into cognitive dissonance is by holding onto an identity that is no longer relevant. For instance, a common case is the man who in younger years did his own car repair, house painting, and remodeling. As time passes, there is less time to do these things, and perhaps, any real inclination. Although he has more money, he is reluctant to give up these activities. His identity is fixed as a "do-it-yourselfer," but that is not the current reality. Sometimes, his home-repair projects remain undone or, if they are completed, it is often at the expense of other fulfilling activities. Likewise, a woman may tend to hold onto the identity of someone who sews most of her clothes long after she discontinues the practice. Her cognitive dissonance and stressful feelings are reinforced every time she passes the pile of fabrics she continues to buy. A graduate student tells a compelling story of cognitive dissonance and self-reflection in the following A Case for Complexity.

A CASE FOR COMPLEXITY

Fresh out of nursing school and recently NCLEX certified, I took a registered nurse (RN) position at a rehabilitation center and realized quickly it was a good decision for me. I was gaining experience, growing more comfortable with the overwhelming responsibility of being a new nurse, and making connections to my education in graduate school. After a few months, however, I was assigned to work as a nurses' aide a few times instead of being given an RN assignment. Considering myself a flexible person and knowing that the facility was suffering a staffing shortage, I made no complaint. My supervisor would often make comments to me, such as "thank you for always being so willing to help," motivating me to just keep quiet. With time, however, my assignment became consistently that of a caregiver and not a nurse. I became frustrated, disappointed, and even sad that I was not being given the opportunity to use my nursing skills and grew to really dislike my job.

Continued

A CASE FOR COMPLEXITY—cont'd

Eventually I started to dread going to work, so I spoke with my supervisor, quoting the number of times I had been assigned to work as an aide. The issue resolved for a few short weeks, then cycled back and I found myself working as an aide for 90 percent of my shifts. One day, barely holding back tears and my patience totally evaporated, I felt I just couldn't do it any longer. I was determined to march to my supervisor's office, file a complaint, and go home for the day. Knowing from experience it wasn't a good idea to act when I was angry, I made an appointment with her for the following week.

The next morning I woke up ill, was laid up in bed, and had a lot of time to think. At first I was angry and felt I was being taken advantage of. In reflecting on the situation over the next several days, however, and in an effort to see things differently, I realized it was a true compliment that management viewed me as a flexible, adaptable employee with an appreciation for the hands-on care that is such an important part of holistic nursing. I came to understand that I couldn't expect my boss to make me happy in my work; I was going to have to find a way to do that myself. I further reflected that it was my choice to go full-time to graduate school and work part-time with a less predictable schedule.

Actively reframing my thoughts helped me approach the conversation with my supervisor from the perspective that I had a lot more to offer than my current position was allowing, and that I wanted to be the very best I could be for my patients. Turns out, she had been thinking the same thing, and was determined to find me a position that would work with my schedule while allowing me to use my skills. She appreciated my approach to the conversation and made it a point to tell me that I was an important part of the organization and truly valued.

I ended up in a position that fit both my needs and the priorities of the facility, all because I was able to step outside of my thoughts for a few days and reframe them into a different perspective. It was very freeing, and helped me successfully approach a very difficult conversation.

—**Emily Fraser Kilroy, BSN, RN**

JOURNAL LEARNING: DISCOVERY, INSIGHT, AND POSSIBLE ACTION

Here and in Chapter 11 are several self-reflective exercises designed to bring your life into clearer focus regarding congruence and possible areas of cognitive dissonance. (See the accompanying *Journal Learning* box.) This process is a form of journal learning. The writing helps to clarify your thoughts and preserve them for future reflection.

JOURNAL LEARNING: FINDING YOUR STATE OF CONGRUENCE

Use the list below to identify your state of congruence at this present moment. Remember that, for most people, congruence is a dynamic state that attains better stability through a long process of self-reflection and life experiences. Once you decide your current state of congruence, reflect on why you reached that conclusion, what your conclusion might mean, and what possible actions you could take in response.

- State 1. I am not sure what I value, and my actions tend to be haphazard and reactive (disorganization).
- State 2. I am not sure what I value, and my actions tend to reflect what others require of me (cognitive dissonance).
- State 3. I know what I value but, for many reasons, my actions do not reflect my values (cognitive dissonance).
- State 4. I know what I value, and my actions reflect my values (congruent).

Journal Learning: Discovery, Insight, and Possible Action

_____

_____

_____

_____

Questions for Reflection

How much of your incongruities or cognitive dissonance may be related to holding on to old identities, past expectations, and outdated images you are still holding onto for yourself? How much is related to living what others see and expect of you? What can be attributed to a need for additional knowledge and skills?

Values clarification exercises are intended to help you with discoveries about your life, work, and values—and to connect those values more closely to the way you lead your life. The exercises are designed to move you through a four-step process of:

- Self-reflection
- Discovery
- Insight
- Possible action

Self-reflection leads to *discovery*. It may come in the form of "I never thought of it that way before" or "That is what has been happening." The next step is *insight*. Insight gives meaning to the discovery. Often, these two stages happen so closely that it may be hard to separate the two. The discovery is the "what is?," and the insight is "what does it mean, and what can I do about it." The last phase is *action*, in which, based on the previous steps, you write down a possible action you will take to actualize your discovery and insight.

Each reading and exercise calls for a pause for self-reflection to uncover your thoughts and feelings. Do not labor in too intellectual a way, but get quiet, and focus on the questions and the answers that arise for you without prolonged pondering. They are the answers of the present moment. Try not to filter them too much through your mind. That can cause too many "oughts" and "shoulds" to emerge. This exercise is to discover the real you, not what others think or what previous conditioning had forged in you the past. Sometimes even humorous and somewhat outrageous thoughts lead to significant discoveries. Think of it as personal brainstorming. Throughout the exercises in chapters 10 and 11, this format is used as a template for your work.

Give yourself the time and the space to reflect in depth. This can be a powerful practice.

First, identify your predominant state of congruent behavior. This may be clearly one over the others, or you may see yourself as having a combination of two (or more). There may be a difference between your assessment of how you behave at work and at home. If so, choose one to start, but eventually consider both. You may have some very enlightening discoveries.

To adopt this process as a practice going forward, obtain a notebook or a special journal for this work dedicated to self-reflection. Life balance is not about doing it all, but doing what is congruent with who you presently are. Jettison the rest, and what is left is not only doable, but can be done with zest and joy.

THE WHEEL OF LIFE

The wheel of life is another exercise by which you can assess the quality of balance in your life at any point in time (Fig. 10-2). The eight spokes of the wheel represent eight components of life that contribute to a full, well-balanced life. This does not mean rigidly attending to each and every component at all times in the same proportion and with the same energy. Balance is a dynamic, not a static, process. There is a natural ebb and flow and a certain amount of chaos in living. But over time, one's actions form a pattern. The wheel serves as a kind of self-reflective compass to check in to see how you are doing and to orient yourself to the whole of life again. Think of it as moving confidently through the various components

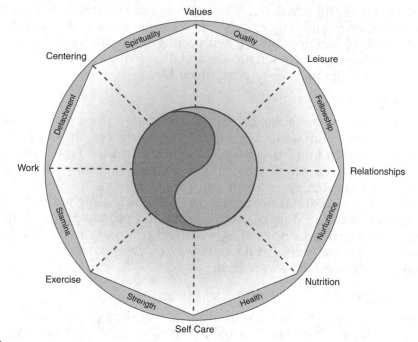

Figure 10-2 The wheel of life.

of your personal and professional life, attending to the various aspects and activities in a manner that is in accordance with your beliefs, values, and goals.

The wheel of life is an orienting tool, a compass. It is not a fixed prescription. Complexity requires moving in and out of order, chaos, and balance, with frequent periods of assessing how one is doing with self-reflective practice.

On the wheel, the four elements noted on the north-south and east-west axes are values, relationships, self-care, and work. These are the primary components to a rich, full life. In a form symbolically reminiscent of the Native American medicine wheel, values reside in the north, representing spirit. Self-care is in the south, grounded in the physical world. Work and relationships occupy the west and east.

Leisure, nutrition, exercise, and centering support the primary components. Between each on the rim of the wheel are the qualities of life you can develop when all components of life are given full measure. These are the rewards for consciously living your life according to your values. As each quality of life is generated, it influences each of the components. This creates an ever-evolving, positive direction for your life. The qualities and practices to develop them are described in depth in Chapter 11.

The center of the wheel signifies balance and congruence: balance as in the image of yin/yang energy and congruence. A congruent person is aware of feelings and acts with authenticity on those feelings. Knowing what your values in life are and then living congruently with those values is the journey to a balanced life.

Values

Your life is ultimately guided and lived by your values. Your values determine how you act in your life. Everything you do in life is a reflection of what you truly believe about life and the way it should be lived. This is true whether or not you are conscious of your values. Time spent on becoming aware of your values and what really matters prepares you to live out those values and to be increasingly congruent. Realization of your values allows purpose and principles to emerge; decisions are clarified, and life flows with less effort. Congruent living reduces your stress and personal tension. You then have more energy for all that wonderfully aware living.

Self-Care

These are the activities related to physical well-being, food, clothing, shelter, and health-promoting behaviors. The goal is to keep your houses in order: body, shelter, and finances.

Work

Work provides meaning and purpose to life and is unique for everyone. Nurses in general feel called to contribute and serve with connection and compassion. Nursing leadership calls to even deeper and wider levels of service, compassion, connection, and empowerment.

Relationships

Relationships provide social and emotional texture. Relationships on the east of the wheel are the complement to work on the west. However, the blending of the east and west is necessary to a fulfilling and balanced life. Successful relationships in your work are essential to complexity leadership, and there is certainly work involved in all relationships.

Exercise and Nutrition

These are essential supports for self-care. Attending to improving your relationships and work without also taking care of your body is very difficult. A healthy body gives you the strength and stamina for your life and work.

Leisure

Activities that have meaning and give you pleasure or a challenge provide balance to your life. They give you a rest from stressful work and a sense of personal satisfaction and accomplishment that you cannot always get from your everyday job. Leisure activities give you opportunities for fellowship as well, building rich relationships.

Centering

While your values influence everything else you do in your life, the practice of centering helps you to uncover those values and gives you the confidence and perspective to follow through on your plans. Centering is a state of optimal relaxation where the mind is clear and the body is calm. Time out and alone to meditate, read inspiring words, or write in a journal is helpful. The more you practice, the easier it is to remain calm and objective in tense situations. Out of these daily periods of quiet and reflection you can clarify your values and sense of spirituality.

Balancing Your Wheel of Life

Refer back to Figure 10-2. Each spoke of the wheel is attached to one component of a balanced, full life. Visualize each spoke as numbered from 1 to 10, with 1 being nearest the hub and representing the least and 10 at the rim and representing the most. Now do the following two-part exercise. You may want to photocopy both the wheel and the *Journal Learning* exercise so you can write freely on them. This exercise works best if you use two different colors of marker or pencil for each part. Clear a time and space with no distractions; then focus and reflect.

When you have completed both parts of the exercise and connected all the dots, you will have formed two patterns that may or may not look similar. Notice your first reaction to the patterns: What do you see? Where are you congruent and where not? For example, if you gave yourself a low number for exercise attention and a low number for exercise satisfaction, then you are congruent in your self-reflection that exercise is a problem for you. You know what needs to be done to change this aspect of your life. Another possible congruent pattern is if you gave yourself a high number for both aspects of exercise, indicating both a high level of congruence and probably good success in that area. The third possibility arises when you see a gap between your level of attention and satisfaction. This can be an indication of cognitive dissonance. A common occurrence is when a person is working many hours, probably with considerable stress, and scores a 9 or 10 for attention but a 2 or 3 for satisfaction. This pattern of being very busy in one life component but without deriving much satisfaction is indicative of cognitive dissonance.

You can see the desirable pattern is to score high numbers on all spokes for both attention and satisfaction. Keep in mind, however, that although this pattern is optimal and may occur on occasion, it is not usual and may in fact be unrealistic. Instead, use the pattern that

JOURNAL LEARNING: BALANCING YOUR WHEEL OF LIFE

Part One
Starting at the top, at *Values,* reflect on each component in turn. Decide how much attention at this present time in your life you are giving to that component. Then choose a number from 1 to 10 that corresponds to that amount of attention, and mark a dot at that point on the wheel. Again, take time to focus and reflect, but avoid over-thinking. Continue around the wheel until you have assessed all eight components. Then connect the dots to form a pattern.

Part Two
Repeat the process using a different color marker, this time assessing how much satisfaction you have with the amount of attention you are paying to each component of your life. Connect those dots. What is your first reaction to your two patterns? What might they mean? What actions do you think you should take?

Journal Learning: Discovery, Insight, and Possible Action

_____

_____

_____

_____

arises at any one time as a compass to orient you to your present circumstances. The following form can help you chart your pattern and discover areas of possible cognitive dissonance as well as reinforce areas of success.

Charting Your Pattern

Use the accompanying *Chart Your Pattern* grid to record your wheel-of-life results. Write down your numbers for attention and satisfaction for each spoke. Then put a check mark in the +C column wherever you have two high numbers (5 to 9) in the attention and satisfaction columns. Put a check mark in the –C column wherever you have two low numbers (1 to 4). Put a check mark in the CD (cognitive dissonance) column wherever you have two widely differing numbers (a span of at least 5). The wider the span, the less congruence and more cognitive dissonance exists in that area. If you have numbers such as 8 and 4 on one spoke, give some thought to whether they should fall in the +C or −C column. If you tend to fall in the middle of the exercise, try to rethink whether your numbers should be a bit closer or farther apart. This is subjective and for you to decide.

You now have an idea about which of the components in your life may be congruent but need attention, which are congruent and successful, and which carry some cognitive dissonance. Think about these scores, and write a few words in the discovery column for each. Transfer the discovery to the journal learning form, and continue with insight and possible actions.

SMALL CHANGES AND BUTTERFLY POWER

When you embark on making changes in your personal or professional life, you are using butterfly power (Briggs and Peat, 1999). Sensitive to initial conditions, in one's personal inner work, even one small action may be amplified throughout a wide system.

Big Ben and a Penny's Worth of Change

The inner workings of London's Big Ben clock is a huge, room-size interplay of gears, weights, pulleys, and a pendulum requiring constant maintenance and calibration. When the technicians check for

CHART YOUR PATTERN

SPOKE	ATTENTION	SATISFACTION	+C	−C	CD	DISCOVERY
VALUES						
LEISURE						
RELATIONSHIPS						
NUTRITION						
SELF-CARE						
EXERCISE						
WORK						
CENTERING						

+C, two higher number (5–9); −C, two lower numbers (1–4); CD, cognitive dissonance (widely differing numbers; a span of at least 5)

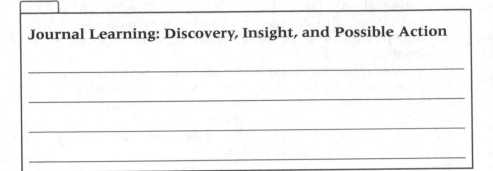

Journal Learning: Discovery, Insight, and Possible Action

accuracy and find Ben off by a few seconds, they employ a very simple solution: a penny or two. The weight of the penny may be enough to bring the clock into perfect balance. This is a fit metaphor for how small actions (butterfly effects) can produce enormous effects. This sensitivity to initial conditions is true for people in their personal and professional lives and within their families and organizations. Small actions and choices do matter. One's physical health benefits from even small efforts: less food, more exercise.

Work flows so much better when you find and fix small snags in the system or work flow. Often answers lie right within the situation. One hospital dealing with an alarming backup and overcrowding in the emergency room researched the system for answers. The usual solution was: if there are more patients, get more physicians and nurses, and expand building space. However, in this instance, it was discovered that a rigid, linear operating room schedule (related to each surgeon having an individualized schedule) caused backups in patient care units, leading to backups in the emergency room; a cascading effect. When the operating room schedule was spread out over the week, the backups were reversed. This was a penny well spent, and many dollars were saved, and patient care service was improved. It must be recognized that there was much skilled relationship work required to help the surgeons to see that simple cause and solution.

In the self-care arena, changing the very small batteries in your smoke alarm can save your home and lives, with enormous results. Drafting a health power of attorney can save so much untold stress and painful dilemmas for families. Relationships are delicate and often turn on small acts of either kindness and forgiveness or thoughtlessness and cruelty. Are your leisure activities consciously chosen or passively self-indulgent? Conscious choice to participate in enjoyable activities may mean the simple act of turning off the television or inviting someone to a social event. Attention to some aspect of centering for even a very brief time regularly can yield specific rewards: stress reduction, calmness, new creative insights, and lower blood pressure. A shift in your values can affect your whole life. Reflecting on what you believe, being true to yourself, shedding old identities, and not living how others think you should release tremendous energy and sense of purpose and passion to make changes.

Awareness, Intention, and Grace

Awareness, intention, and grace are three attributes that can help you make a difference with your small changes. Being consciously aware rather than living on automatic can stop you from speaking out without first thinking about how your words will affect others. Intention gives focus to passion. While one needs to be passionate to make creative change in one's life, it is intention that makes things happen. Laura Day writes in her book *The Circle* (2001) that your intentionality is your will: "Your will organizes and mobilizes all the other energies inside of you and around you into an irresistible force. Your ability to make a choice and to stick with it—your will—is your most powerful inner resource" (p. 15). Ralph Blum (1982) describes people not as doers, but as deciders. Once your decision is clear, the doing becomes effortless.

The third attribute is grace. Grace is a manner in which you move through life more easily on a daily basis. It includes being open to new experiences without prejudgment, staying centered in difficult situations, and acting with kindness, love, and joy. With awareness, intention and grace, you can be an attractor, that pattern of energy that attracts more energy to it. People are drawn to and want to give to those who live with awareness, intention, and grace. Big Ben is a complicated mechanism. But so, too, are human beings: a complex web of interactions and relationships that is very sensitive to individual choices and actions.

SUMMARY

The complexity leader employs personal being and awareness to work toward congruence and reduce cognitive dissonance. Personal and professional life balance can be assessed and adjusted through self-reflection and attention to important life components. Chapter 11 provides additional opportunities for self-reflection and journal learning.

QUESTIONS FOR SELF-REFLECTION

1. What small influence do I have in my work situation? What "pennies" do I have to spend and how can I use them appropriately?
2. What leadership issue is keeping me from moving toward more congruence?

3. What are the areas of cognitive dissonance to which I will set my intention?

Self-Reflection: What Have I Learned?

_____

_____

_____

_____

_____

10–1   CRITICAL THINKING QUESTION

The complexity leader is congruent, both in thoughts, feelings, and behaviors and in knowledge of complex adaptive systems, leadership style, and actions and personal being and awareness. From your experience, describe one leader with whom you have worked that is either congruent or not and describe this person's behavior and impact on others.

10–2   CRITICAL THINKING CASE FOR COMPLEXITY

I am a unit-based nursing educator, and in this role I have seen certified nursing assistants (CNAs) struggle with the demands of their work. Here is Nancy's story, which is representative of many in her position. I set out to improve the work environment for Nancy and her colleagues by employing complexity principles. These actions are described as well.

Nancy has been a nursing assistant on the adult oncology unit for over 7 years. Nancy loves her work as a nursing assistant, but she is very concerned about recent events. The unit has been in a period of transition with an interim nurse manager who is relatively new to the institution. Although there are several experienced nurses on the unit, most of them were hired after Nancy, and Nancy is not sure whom she can trust. She is getting tired of all of the changes, and she is skeptical about the new nurses who are younger than her own daughter. To make matters worse, rumors are flying about the candidates for the nurse manager position, and it is difficult to know fact from fiction. Nancy has attended staff meetings and heard about patient satisfaction scores, quality initiatives, and budget concerns, but what do those have to do with her?

It was a typical 12-hour workday, and Nancy had a seven-patient assignment. Morning report was always a challenge. With "Partnership Rounding," the nurses gave report at the bedside, but Nancy was working with two nurses today, which meant that she would miss part of report. She decided to take report with Jess, and she would have to catch up with Meghan later. The problem was that one of Meghan's patients had to be transferred to the special care unit, so Nancy would not get Meghan's report until later in the morning. That was typical; the nurses never seemed to have the time to keep Nancy updated. Luckily, Nancy had seen the night certified nursing assistant (CNA) and got a brief update.

Nancy's morning routine included daily weights, morning baths, helping her patients order breakfast, and obtaining blood glucose testing and vital signs. She had a patient on strict bed rest and another who was recovering from abdominal surgery. Patients were calling for assistance to the bathroom, and she was being paged to get someone on a stretcher for a CT scan. She looked around for help, but the nurses said they were too busy. It infuriated Nancy to see one of the nurses take a seat at the desk and sign on to the computer.

Training programs for CNAs provide a total of 150 hours of classroom, skills laboratory, and supervised clinical practice. CNAs learn the necessary skills to perform tasks under the direct supervision of a registered nurse, but their linear training does not necessarily prepare them to practice in a complex adaptive system such as an adult oncology unit in an acute care setting. Although much has been done to provide a thorough orientation program and continuing education for registered nurses, the nursing assistant is expected to complete orientation within 2 to 3 weeks, with fewer continuing education opportunities. Meanwhile, nurses are busy, and supporting the nursing assistants is often low on the priority hierarchy. The result is that the nursing assistants are frustrated and angry with the system and with the registered nurses. They feel alienated from the team and begin to operate as a shadow system. Gossip, rumors, decreased patient satisfaction scores, and quality issues become a problem.

As a unit-based educator, I am responsible for providing education for all of the nursing staff on the adult oncology unit. The challenge is finding the time and commitment from everyone on the unit to support education for nursing assistants. I brought my concerns to our unit leadership team, which provided the support I needed to create a Nursing Assistant Practice and Quality Council. The goals for the council were to provide support, leadership, and education for our nursing assistants. We scheduled our first meeting, and I sent an e-mail announcement, promoted the council to the core group of nursing assistants, and asked one of our staff nurses to partner with me in leading the group. Every nursing assistant was encouraged to attend, with the promise that they would be paid if they came in on their day off, and they would be expected to attend if they were scheduled to work during the time of the meeting.

The first meeting was well attended. The group decided on the meeting schedule that day. Asking questions has been helpful in solving some of the difficult issues that arise from our work: how can we deal with patient satisfaction scores, the supply budget, and making partnership rounding work for nursing assistants?

As the leader for the Nursing Assistant Practice and Quality Council, I begin by listening actively to questions and concerns that are brought to the group and by providing minimum specifications and simple rules such as the patient satisfaction survey and balanced scorecard results. Generative relationships have begun to form, with new ideas and strategies for solving some of our most challenging issues. New practice initiatives are presented along with education that is directed specifically toward the role of the nursing assistant. A recent example is the glycemic control protocol, which includes checking the patient's blood glucose prior to meals along with carbohydrate counting. The protocol is a particular challenge for our unit because our patient population has a meal service that delivers food only on request. The nursing assistants were full collaborators in learning the procedures and in deciding how they would carry them out. They saw their role as partnering with the patients.

Complexity science helps us understand that nursing units are complex adaptive systems. Viewing the system through the lens of complexity, we see that coaching and training the team to work together and involving others in the process is part of building a better complex system. A vision, such as providing the group with minimum specifications, allows the group to self-organize, with new behaviors emerging from the group rather than having rules imposed on it. In allowing the group to find its own solutions, I have found that members' commitment to the unit and their practice has become stronger, and they have emerged as a team. Recognizing and listening to the shadow system has helped us identify problems and concerns and allowed us the opportunity to use the shadow system to provide accurate and timely information. Furthermore, a trusting and supportive relationship has formed among all members of the practice council, including the staff nurse and unit-based educator.

Diane D. Vachon, RN, OCN

10–3   CRITICAL THINKING QUESTION ▆▆▆▆▆

The nurse educator embodies qualities and actions of the complexity leader as well as congruence. Identify some of these qualities. What are some of the indicators that Nancy was in cognitive dissonance? How did the educator help move Nancy and her colleagues toward congruence?

REFERENCES

Beck, J.D., & Yeager, N.M. (2001). *The leader's window: Mastering the four styles of leadership to build high-performing teams* (2nd ed.). Boston: Nicholas Brealey Publishing.

Benner, P. (1984). *From novice to expert: Excellence and power in clinical nursing practice.* Addison Wesley Publishing Company.

Blum, R.H. (1982/2008). *The book of runes.* New York: Thomas Dunne Books/ St. Martin's Press.

Briggs, J., & Peat, F.D. (1999). *Seven life lessons of chaos: Timeless wisdom from the science of change.* New York: HarperCollins.

Day, L. (2001). *The circle.* New York: Jeremy Tarcher.

Festinger, L. (1957). *A theory of cognitive dissonance.* Stanford, CA: Stanford University Press.

Heermann, B. (2004). *Noble purpose: Igniting extraordinary passion for life and work.* Fairfax, VA: QSU Publishing Company.

Rogers, C.R. (1961/2004). *On becoming a person: A therapist's view of psychotherapy.* London: Constable.

11

SELF-REFLECTIVE PRACTICES FOR PERSONAL BEING AND AWARENESS

Sensitive to initial conditions, each choice you make, each step you take, may be just one more in your current direction. But it could very well be the one that ripples across the rest of your life.

INTRODUCTION

This chapter expands on the balanced wheel of life to include the qualities that can be generated on attending to important components of personal and professional life. For review, the eight components of the wheel are: values, relationships, self-care, work, leisure, nutrition, exercise, and centering (see the wheel of life illustration in Chapter 10). The following qualities are generated: quality, fellowship, nurturance, health, strength, stamina, detachment, and spirituality. You become increasingly congruent as well.

QUALITIES ON THE WHEEL OF LIFE

The qualities on the wheel of life are generated by living a dynamically balanced and congruent life. The eight qualities are placed strategically around the wheel to illustrate the rewards that are possible from practicing and attending to particular aspects of life. However, the qualities are not only rewards; they also serve as catalysts for further growth and positive change. For example, on either side of the *work* spoke are *detachment* and *stamina*, two very important qualities to support you in your daily work, whether with the demands of leadership or a robust home life. A practice of centering promotes detachment, and stamina is developed by regular exercise.

The practice of centering brings forth spirituality that directly influences the realization of your values. What you consider to be a quality life is based on your own ideas and interpretation. Living congruently helps you achieve what you consider to be a quality life.

In your leisure life, a value-driven outlook fosters leisure activities that are particular to you. For leisure activities of a social nature, fellowship is enhanced as you take part in activities with others and form meaningful relationships. Nurturance is the social and family function of caring for others. Nurturance is given and received through acts of kindness and service activities. Nurturance is a trait of leadership seldom recognized but important to all human relationships. Nursing leaders, especially, have the opportunity to transfer their inherent caring stance into leadership for true congruence.

Attention to nutrition and self-care practices leads to the quality of general health and well-being, just as the quality of strength is the benefit of self-care and exercise. Stamina, essential to busy professional and home lives, is also the result of exercise. Complexity leaders are role models who inspire best when not fatigued and are able to both physically and emotionally persevere through difficult and hectic times.

Another quality so vital for life and work is detachment. Detachment can be likened to objectivity but is more encompassing. It is acting according to beliefs, values, purpose, and even passion, but at the same time not being attached to the outcome of the effort. Differentiation is a form of detachment in which one knows and truly expresses one's views without being caught up and anxious about others expressing theirs.

Centering is the primary practice for developing detachment. Setting time aside for reflection, meditation journaling, or reading inspiring words are examples of centering. As the capacity is deepened to stay calm physiologically, this transfers to potentially tense situations, and life can be approached with a more reflective mindset. Nurse leaders who participated in mindfulness meditation classes were found to have decreases in stress, depression, and anxiety.

Pipe and colleagues (2009) conducted a study with nurse leaders to determine the effectiveness of a mindfulness meditation program for stress management. They discovered at the beginning and early stages of the project that, for the total sample (control and treatment group), the intensity and prevalence of stress was much greater than those in the general population. This is a clear demonstration of the demanding roles and lives nurse leaders have. The intervention, teaching Mindfulness Meditation to these nurse leaders, was intended to help them deepen their capacity for attention and to strengthen present-moment awareness. Based on Jean Watson's Theory of Human Caring, the researchers assumed that nurturing themselves by mindfulness meditation would extend to their being more caring and nurturing of others. The researchers believed that the ability to be fully present with others and with emerging situations would lead to more effective leadership, including teamwork, communication, and decision making, all desirable traits of the complexity leader. Results of the study were significantly positive. The participants reported reduced stress, depression, and anxiety for themselves and in relationship to the control group. Mindfulness meditation can be a supportive practice for personal being and awareness.

The exercise in the accompanying Journal Learning feature will help you assess the overall pattern of qualities in your life. Think about each quality in your present life and then, for each quality, give yourself a 1 to 10 (10 being best) by circling the number for each quality and then connecting the circles vertically.

PERSONAL CHANGE

There is an assumption that when you assess your life balance and quality, you will want to make the changes you identified so you can be that complexity leader: the one who has a balanced and exciting but less stressful personal and professional life. However, embarking on new behaviors entails moving with discipline and some level of risk out of your comfort zone (for example, see *A Case For Complexity*).

Risk is about taking action, behaving or speaking by conscious choice because you believe it is best for you and others and is congruent with your vision, values, and principles. What keeps people from taking risks? It can stem from two sources: either fear and anxiety or inertia. For example, in *A Case for Complexity,* Sara's hesitation at the conference probably was due more to fear and anxiety with some cognitive dissonance (who was she to think she could participate with all those important people?), but with her fatigue there was certainly some inertia, too.

Not risking because of fear and anxiety is related to trust, trusting yourself and in the goodness of others. It is trust that when you act in accordance with your vision, values, and principles (congruently), you will be safe and might even receive rewards beyond your expectations.

These words by the 13th century poet Rumi (Barks, 1995) illustrate trust, risk, and reward.

Birds make great sky-circles of their freedom.
How do they learn it?
They fall, and falling, they are given wings.

CHART YOUR QUALITIES OF LIFE PATTERN

1	2	3	4	5	QUALITY	6	7	8	9	10
1	2	3	4	5	FELLOWSHIP	6	7	8	9	10
1	2	3	4	5	NURTURANCE	6	7	8	9	10
1	2	3	4	5	HEALTH	6	7	8	9	10
1	2	3	4	5	STRENGTH	6	7	8	9	10
1	2	3	4	5	STAMINA	6	7	8	9	10
1	2	3	4	5	DETACHMENT	6	7	8	9	10
1	2	3	4	5	SPIRITUALITY	6	7	8	9	10

Journal Learning: Discovery, Insight, and Possible Action

What is your pattern? What are your discoveries, insights, and possible actions?

_____

_____

_____

_____

_____

A CASE FOR COMPLEXITY

Sara sat that morning in the large hotel conference center with several hundred others at the big leadership conference. She had invested 24 hours of travel and a great deal of money to be there. With only 3 hours sleep, she listened drowsily to the opening remarks. One of the conference moderators asked for volunteers to learn about and then facilitate discussion groups called Conversation Cafes. Through her sleepy haze she realized that this was something she wanted to do, but she was tired. At the same time, she thought, "Wait a minute! You went to school, learned about and teach this; you consider yourself a leader, and you just sit there?" And her hand shot up! At that moment she envisioned a distinct image of stepping into a circle, as if she were stepping into that vision she held of herself. It was if she were stepping into her own congruence. Sara's risk was very well rewarded. She sat at lunch with the hosts and learned from the very authors whose work inspired her to attend. That action, that risk, transformed what would have been a pleasant but passive event into a rich experience.

Trust that when you step into a situation, your own congruence will be the wind that supports you. The other aspect of risk is overcoming the inertia to change an aspect of yourself. It is a risk because you are leaving your comfort zone to endure some level of discomfort or hardship in order to improve a condition such as your health or a living situation. You may have only a faint glimpse of the possible reward for your effort. Whereas trust is the key to overcoming fear, discipline is the key to overcoming inertia. The more firmly formed your vision of the end result is, the easier discipline becomes.

Leap into congruence!

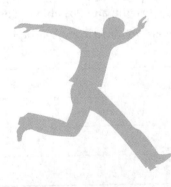

Trust and discipline can reinforce each other. Trust that you are living your best self and that with disciplined effort you will grow into more of who you want to be. Discipline does take some trust to leap into action. Each act of discipline brings you further along in your journey. David Lloyd George (Hayward, 1987) encourages discipline and risk with his version of "just do it." He encourages people to not be afraid to take a big step if one is indicated because you cannot cross a chasm in two small steps.

When you find yourself hesitating to take a risk, sort out for yourself whether it is related to fear and anxiety or not wanting to move out of your comfort zone. If it is fear, trust is easier when you are consciously aware of your own values and beliefs. With self-reflection, check in with yourself to be clear. However, if you discover that a great deal of your hesitancy is really about wanting to stay comfortable, hold out before you your vision of the new change, challenge, and adventure and the reward that waits for you. Risk takes trust and discipline in order for you to be the leader of your own congruent life and ultimately becoming a complexity leader.

Beach Reverie

I step out onto the stony beach
They call me, these stones
Pick me! Pick me!
I reach out, scoop up, and cradle in my palm
One
Gray, white, striped, oval
I am overcome by its alluring smoothness caressing my hand
This smoothness announces the stone's
Long-long life journey
From sharp and jagged to ocean-washed silken skin
It tells me of tumbles and trials
Efforts to hold on
Then, moments of surrender
"What happens will happen"
Such a role model, this stone
My wish....
To become this gray/white silken smoothness
To live in such a manner where jagged edges are washed smooth
By the surf of a life lived
With challenge, adventure, vision and effort
Till I am receptive, reflective, calm and still
Tumbled to silken, smooth peace

—D.C.

THE SELF-CARE SPECTRUM

Two areas require discussion in more detail. The first is the self-care spectrum, the grounded physical aspects of being that include self-care, nutrition, and exercise in the south of the wheel. The second is the process that is less quantifiable, more abstract, but no less important: mind and spirit, and centering to cultivate detachment and spirituality.

The wheel of life, with its eight components and qualities, can be a powerful model for assessing your overall life. Occasionally, people look at the wheel of life and all the aspects of their lives and, feeling overwhelmed, wonder "Where do I start?" A good place to start is approaching change in an "inside-out" manner. That is, by starting with self-care. Self-care is about getting your "houses" in order: the houses of your body, shelter, and finances. Are you overdue for your dental checkup? Is your garage full of everything but the car? Are important papers scattered and hard to find? Do you have a will? Is it time to be saving for college? Do you need to do estate and retirement planning? These things are in your control.

Self-care is in your control. In areas of work and relationships, there can be a tendency to cast the control to others—in work, "If this were a better place to work..." and in relationships, "If they would do better...." Start with those things nearest to you and really in your control. Covey (1989) speaks about the circle of influence and circle of concern. When you focus on trying to fix those things not under your control, you are reactive and not able to have much influence; as your focus stays "out there" (concern), your influence over events decreases. If, however, you work on those things close by and within your control in a proactive way, your circle of influence increases, and your circle of concern decreases; thus, you can then effect change in a wider sphere. The sense of accomplishment from succeeding at changing a behavior or circumstance carries over into other parts of your life. You feel good, releasing new energy. This energy acts as a leverage point for further positive action. So how do you get your houses in order?

The first house of self-care is your body: health and life insurance, smoke alarms, seat belts, regular dental checkups, updated eyeglass prescriptions, keeping informed about health-care advances, taking medications properly, asking questions of your health-care providers. Exercise and nutrition are part of self-care as well. The second house is shelter—your home: clean, ordered, repaired, uncluttered, harmonious, safe, welcoming. The third house is finance: living within your means, savings, investments, wills, retirement planning, using awareness and choice when spending money, acquiring knowledge through books and newspapers, seeking professional counsel.

Disorder in self-care is a real energy drainer. Every time you look at or are reminded of an uncompleted repair, appointment not made, or clutter taking over your living space, you are draining energy away. Take an inventory of your three houses. What items come to the top of the list? While developing the list may seem daunting in itself, it can show what is within your circle of influence. Then start very small. Take one item from each house for a start. For example, schedule one doctor's appointment. The call takes a very few minutes, but you will feel that sense of accomplishment from getting that done. Then select one corner of clutter, drawer, or closet to tackle. Each small job done is a success. Buy a book on financial matters to check up on how you are doing. Then you can decide whether to seek professional advice. You do not have to be rich to profit from good financial advice. Many times a first consultation is free.

It is amazing how working on one area of self-care influences other areas. For example, you may choose to cut down on the number of times you eat out in a week and buy simple, healthy ingredients to cook at home. You will save a substantial amount of money not spent in restaurants and get healthier at the same time. Giving clothes and household items that you no longer use to a charity unclutters your house, and you can take an itemized deduction on your income tax as well. Each task done boosts your sense of accomplishment, control, and energy. So many of these projects take very little time in actual minutes. It is all the thoughts of tackling them that take hours. Time management is a component and ally of self-care activities. One less hour of television frees time for one more self-care success. Each small success builds a better day, day by day.

As you start to see progress in your three houses of self-care, you build confidence in your ability to be effective in other areas of your life. Increased energy will help you take on exercise and time out for centering practices. Your circle of influence will expand to include work and relationships. Your houses of body, shelter, and finance will be outward demonstrations of your values and your self. Now do some journal learning using the accompanying form.

The House of Your Body and the Mind-Body Connection

Exercise and good nutrition are the mainstays of a healthy body. It is easy to forget how a healthy strong body is the key to calm, energetic, meaningful work and a rich relationship-filled life. Seek out a health club or gym to start an exercise program if you do not already do so.

It cannot be emphasized enough how strong the mind-body connection is. There are two routes to becoming anxious: mind to body and body to mind. The following is a very simplified explanation for a complex biochemical process that occurs all the time.

JOURNAL LEARNING: SHELTER AND FINANCES

Shelter

Think of your house or, better yet, walk through it with a critical eye assessing for clutter, cleanliness, repairs, organization, peacefulness, and so on. Does your house reflect who you are, and is it congruent with your values? Write down your discoveries, insights, and possible actions. Consider repeating this process for your work space or office.

Journal Learning: Discovery, Insight, and Possible Action

_____

_____

_____

_____

Finances

Consider your finances. Are you living within your means? Are your financial records in order? How do you stand regarding financial planning for college, retirement, and estate issues? Where are your problem areas? What information do you need to put order and organization into your financial life?

Journal Learning: Discovery, Insight, and Possible Action

_____

_____

_____

_____

Mind-Body Connection

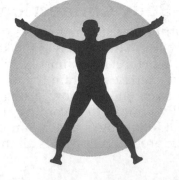

Mind to Body

Thoughts precede feelings. In his cognitive therapy work, Ellis (1987) describes how, first, there is an event, and, second, a person interprets the event (thoughts). Based on the thought, there are emotions. Ellis says interpretation of events can be reframed, calling it cognitive reframing. In other words, interpreting the event in a more positive way (changing your thought), will change your feelings about the event. This is not denial, but realistically assessing the situation to a more positive interpretation. This will help you and your body to remain calmer and more focused. You will have fewer of the anxiety symptoms of racing heart, sweating, and dry mouth associated with anxiety.

Body to Mind

The condition of one's body on a day-to-day basis affects one's thoughts and feelings. Not eating breakfast and having low blood sugar, not feeling well, or being out of condition whereby you easily get short of breath may create some of the same feelings (physically) that you have in anxiety or feeling nervous. For example, you may attend a meeting that normally does not make you anxious. But this day you skipped breakfast and only drank some strong caffeinated coffee. You are setting yourself up for feelings that mimic anxiety, when you are really on the "caffeine high, sugar low" rollercoaster. A negative cycle can happen in either direction. For balance, you need healthy, positive thoughts and a healthy, well-exercised and well-nourished body. Any improvement you make in either of these will pay back enormously, and you will see and feel the difference very soon after you start to change your exercise and eating habits. Stamina and strength are yours as well to keep going with some equanimity.

The following is a self-care quiz that covers many aspects of self-care. Use the journal learning portion to help you see where you are doing well and where you can improve. Although the most points you can score is 100, there is no average or best score. The best plan is to try to better your current score over time. If you just returned from an overeating vacation, you may want to wait until you are in a more regular activity pattern to take this quiz.

Cultivating Detachment and Spirituality With Centering Practices

Watts (1995) quotes Chuang-Tzu as saying, "The perfect man employs his mind as a mirror; it grasps nothing, it refuses nothing, it receives, but does not keep" (p. 21). Watts continues to describe detachment as "having no regrets for the past, no fears for the future, to neither prolong the stay of things pleasant, nor hasten the departure of things unpleasant." Another aspect of detachment is suspending judgment of

A. In the last 3 days, I:

Exercised (aerobic or strength training)	Y/N
Set aside quiet time for reflection/inspirational reading	Y/N
Watched fewer than 6 hours of television	Y/N

SCORE _____ Each YES = +5; Each NO = −5

B.

I consistently use my seat belt in the car	Y/N
I have a smoke alarm in my house	Y/N
I have had a massage or other body work	Y/N

SCORE _____ Each YES = +5; Each NO = −5

C. In the last 48 hours I ate/drank:

1 or more donuts	Y/N
More than 4 cups of coffee	Y/N
1 or more sodas (even diet)	Y/N
Cream sauce	Y/N
Restaurant fast food (other than salad)	Y/N

SCORE _____ Each NO = +5; Each YES = −5

Oatmeal	Y/N
A soy product	Y/N
At least 4 fruits	Y/N
At least 4 vegetables	Y/N

SCORE _____ Each YES = +5; Each NO = −5

D. I know my:

Blood pressure	Y/N
Cholesterol level (total)	Y/N

SCORE _____ Each YES = +5; Each NO = −5

E. In the past year, I had a (if applicable; if not, mark Yes):

Physical examination	Y/N
Mammogram/prostate examination	Y/N
Dental examination	Y/N

SCORE _____ Each YES = +5; Each NO = −5

TOTAL SCORE (A+ B+C+D+E) = _____ **Highest possible score is 100**

Journal Learning: Discovery, Insight, and Possible Action

_____

_____

_____

_____

_____

bad or good about situations or persons and just seeing them as they are. There is an observer quality about having a sense of detachment. When leading a group, be a weather reporter. Rather than giving your opinion, comment on what you observe, what is going on. This allows the conversation to emerge instead of trying to steer it. While that may seem to take up too much time, this letting go of the outcome, this detachment, frequently leads to better outcomes and faster conclusions in the long run (Mindell, 1995).

One practical way to realize you are gaining the quality of detachment in your life is when something or someone who usually annoys you, causing you to react automatically, no longer provokes that response in you. Does this mean giving up being passionate? No; passions, excitement, and strong beliefs are the greatest motivations for living. A complexity leader lives the paradox of passion and detachment every day.

How do you manage detachment? Detachment just emerges, often subtly and over time, as you attend to other aspects of your life. While a centering practice is key to developing detachment, attention to other areas of life has great influence. All self-care activities—eating well, exercising, having your houses in order, reducing cognitive dissonance, and being increasingly congruent—prepare you for experiencing detachment.

During your day, there are ways to work toward detachment. Hanh (1991) suggests using those situations that annoy you, such as red lights and ringing phones, as signals to practice. When these annoying situations occur, breathe in, smile out. There are so many inactive moments in which you can practice being present in order to promote detachment: watching the shampoo slowly ooze into your hand, waiting for the red light to change, waiting for the microwave to finish, waiting for the Internet download, waiting at the copy machine, and waiting in line. You can choose how to react in those moments. You can be present, receptive, and breathe calmly, or you can tense up impatiently. In time, these periods composed of inactive moments can coalesce into a detachment way of life. Wilde (1994) has a phrase to describe a nonjudgmental "being in the present" attitude: if you are caught in the rain, do rain.

In *A Course in Miracles* (1985), a most helpful thought when a potentially upsetting event occurs is to think that there may be another way to look at this event. An affirmation by Paramahansa Yogananda (1982) describes living daily with a sense of detachment. This affirmation is an excellent example of the "being in flow": "I will be calmly active, actively calm. I will not become lazy and mentally ossified. Nor will I be overactive, able to earn money but unable to enjoy life. I will meditate regularly to maintain true balance" (p. 90).

Centering

Centering encompasses many practices that are intended to prepare you to deal with the difficulties, uncertainties, and challenges in work and life with a calm, quiet center, certain about yourself if not the circumstances. Centering keeps you in touch with ideas and perspectives greater than your own yearnings and needs.

There is a wide range of centering practices that can meet individual preferences. These include meditation, reading, journaling, affirmations, walking, going into nature, deep breathing, yoga, tai chi, and other stretching or rhythmic exercise. Even a ritual of tea or coffee at the same time every day, sitting quietly in a contemplative state, is a form of centering. See Table 11–1, *10 Methods of Centering*. Also see the annotated bibliography (see Appendix).

Table 11–1	10 METHODS OF CENTERING
PRACTICE	**DESCRIPTION**
Meditation	Set aside time each day—such as early morning—to sit in silence and clear your mind. When thoughts come in, keep coming back to the present silent moment. Even 5 or 10 minutes, done regularly, can be effective. Take a class, or read a book for instruction.
Reading	Reading inspirational words, poetry, or self-help books has a positive effect on the nervous system and provides an uplifting focus for your thoughts.
Journaling	A most effective self-reflection practice is writing down daily thoughts and aspirations for discovery and insight.
Affirmations	Reading and writing affirmations induces positive energy and keeps you focused on the present moment. Choose and frame a favorite affirmation, and place it in your work area where you can see and read it often.
Breathing	Deep, slow breathing into the abdomen practiced with meditation quiets the mind, slows the pulse, and lowers blood pressure. Once integrated into your practice, you can stop and breathe before difficult conversations or when in tense situations.
Yoga, tai chi	Both yoga and tai chi combine stretching and movements that require the practice of presence.
Prayer	Prayer inspires and brings focus to those who find comfort in practicing their faith.

Table 11–1	10 METHODS OF CENTERING—cont'd

PRACTICE	DESCRIPTION
Music	Classical, Celtic, New Age, or chanting are some forms of music that focus, calm, or inspire. Choose and play music that brings you back to your center.
Connect with nature	Find a park, trail, hilltop, water's edge, or garden that connects you to the natural world, and visit regularly to refresh and renew.
Anchoring object	Choose a stone, crystal, art work, or other special object to place in your work area to remind you to breathe, focus, and center. A very small object can be carried in your pocket to use as a touchstone in times of stress.

The *Tao Te Ching* (1992, p. 24) encapsulates the beliefs, traits, and practices of the complexity leader who embodies personal being and awareness. For example:

He who stands on tip toe doesn't stand firm.
He who rushes ahead, doesn't go far.
He who tries to shine, dims his own light.
He who defines himself can't know who he really is.
He who has power over others can't empower himself.
He who clings to his work will create nothing that endures.
If you want to be in accord with the Tao, just do your job, then
    let go.

SUMMARY

Personal being and awareness are enhanced through self-reflection and journal learning. Centering practices help the complexity leader to remain calm and present, even in disruptive and challenging circumstances. The complexity leader is balanced in mind, body, and spirit, ever evolving toward greater congruence. In Chapter 12, you will have the opportunity to assess your complexity leadership knowledge and determine your complexity leadership profile.

QUESTIONS FOR SELF-REFLECTION

1. What self-reflective practice can I start that will enhance my sense of detachment?
2. How can I become more comfortable with disorder, conflict, and disruption?

3. How satisfied am I with my current centering practice? What is my next step?

Self-Reflection: What Have I Learned?

_____

_____

_____

_____

_____

11–1   CRITICAL THINKING QUESTION ▰▰▰▰

Steven Covey's Circle of Influence and Circle of Concern are discussed in this chapter. Think of a situation that seems out of control in which you can identify your circle of influence rather than focus on your circle of concern and describe this.

11–2   CRITICAL THINKING CASE
FOR COMPLEXITY ▰▰▰▰

It is essential to first keep peace within yourself; then you can also bring peace to others. I have the courage to share my story about achieving harmony within my body, mind, spirit, and community. Many nurses ignore their own health. The assumption is that nurses interpret their nursing knowledge and apply it to their own health. While this may lead nurses to better care for others, something is seriously amiss in many nurses when caring for themselves. I was one nurse who failed to interpret my understanding of health to my own life.

I am a product of the nursing education of the 1950s, educated in the framework that looked at the human being as a bio-psycho-social and spiritual being. My courage was first to see in a mirror that I was overweight. The nursing knowledge I used to solve this problem came from this overarching framework of holism. The solution, which I had used to counsel my patients, was elegant in its simplicity—to take small steps to lose weight and to incorporate an understanding of the impact of physical, social, and spiritual wellness into these steps.

I identified the concept of "harmony" as the essential philosophy for creating a healthy self. This harmony was an encompassing understanding of body, mind, spirit, and community. Using the nursing process, I made weekly changes. I made changes in my diet, exercise, fluid intake, and in how I responded to situations. When evaluated, these changes brought successes in some weeks and not in others. Overall, I lost more than 170 pounds without gastric bypass or band surgery.

As I achieved success in harmonizing my body, mind, and spirit, I sought to extend this harmony into my relationship to my nursing community. I enrolled in a recent summer graduate course to improve my spiritual sense of community. I learned that, as one nurse, I can make a small change that impacts the community.

In a short but intense time, through relationships with other nurses (these small steps), we formed our community, and I learned about the complexity science paradigm view with the emphasis on relationships between dynamic beings, rather than on the beings themselves. During the course, students shared their stories. We created harmony as we took care of ourselves in the group. This extension of the effectiveness of the personal to the interpersonal was the final small step needed to transform my lessons from others to self and back to others. The nourishing of others through relationships is a powerful means of integrating the concept of harmony from a personal focus to an interpersonal one. The lessons from this work will ultimately enhance our ability to care for our patients, their loved ones, and ourselves.

Anne M. Logan, RN, MHSA, BSN, RAC-CT

11–3   CRITICAL THINKING QUESTION

What characteristics of balance and self-care does this nurse exemplify? What lesson might you learn from her story?

REFERENCES

Barks, C. (1995). *The essential Rumi*. San Francisco: Harper.
Covey, S.R. (1989). *The 7 habits of highly effective people*. New York: Simon & Schuster.
Ellis, A., & Windy, D. (1987/2007). *The practice of rational emotive behavior therapy* (2nd ed.). New York, Springer.
Foundation for Inner Peace. (1985). *A course in miracles*. Tiburon, CA: Author.
Hanh, Thich Nhat. (1991). *Peace is every step: The path of mindfulness in everyday life*. New York: Bantam Books.
Hayward, S. (1987/1999). *Begin it now* (2nd ed.). Australia: Hayward Books.
Mindell, A. (1995). *Sitting in the fire: Large group transformation using conflict and diversity*. Portland, OR: Lao Tse Press.
Mitchell, S. (1992). *Tao te ching*. New York: Harper Perennial.
Pipe, T.B., Bortz, J.J., Dueck, A., et al. (2009). Nurse leader mindfulness meditation program for stress management: A randomized controlled trial. *J Nurs Adm, 39*(3), 130-137.
Watts, A.W. (1995). *Become what you are*. Boston: Shambhala Publications.
Wilde, S. (1994). *Weight loss for the mind*. New York: Hay House.
Yogananda, P. (1982). *Metaphysical meditations*. Los Angeles: Self-Realization Fellowship.

12

THE CALL FOR COMPLEXITY LEADERSHIP

Complexity leaders are attractors. With new ideas and ways of leading, they create their own butterfly effects.

■ OBJECTIVES

- Apply the concepts of complexity leadership to health-care delivery.
- Describe the developmental process to transformational and then to complexity leadership.
- Assess your level of knowledge, actions, and practices with the complexity leadership profile.
- Discuss the relationship between complexity leadership and graduate nursing leadership roles.

INTRODUCTION

With the complexity leadership model as the framework, this book has explored health-care organizations as complex adaptive systems, surveyed the history of leadership theory, and highlighted contemporary leadership styles and practices. Current applications of complexity science concepts to research and practice in health care were examined. The third and essential component of complexity leadership—personal being and awareness—provided opportunities for self-reflection for personal growth. This final chapter reviews the key themes of the three units and discusses the developmental process that leads toward complexity leadership. A valuable feature is the *Complexity Leadership Profile* self-assessment, in which you can determine your level of knowledge understanding and application of the complexity leadership model.

COMPLEXITY SCIENCE CONCEPTS AND HEALTH-CARE ORGANIZATIONS

A complexity perspective toward health-care organizations dramatically shifts a leader's worldview from reporting lines, boxes, or detailed strategic plans to distributed control, local solutions, and webs of relationship. The top-down, plan, organize, control, and direct approach is replaced with a more organic, dynamic process of connections, and on occasion, surprises. The vibrancy of a health-care organization is not just seen at the senior leadership level but can be validated at the edge, at local, point of service sites. When hospitals seeking Magnet Recognition are appraised, although the role of the chief nursing officer is important to creating the environment, the direct-care nurses across the organizations are the ones who reveal the true nature of the organization. When nurses at the unit level are empowered through self-governance and interdisciplinary support to be decision makers in the interest of best care, and they perceive themselves to be both autonomous and interdependent, they embody the Magnet ideal. Magnet hospitals are examples of self-organizing systems at their best.

Complexity science applied to health care is not just theoretical anymore. The microsystems studies and models by the Dartmouth group have widespread influence in health-care practice and quality improvement initiatives. Anderson's evidence that the quality of communication and relationships corresponds to the quality of resident outcomes in nursing homes is changing the way nursing home management is practiced. The complexity of nurses' work being investigated by Ebright and her colleagues explains the details of the work, but of more value is the evidence for others to see how complex, challenging, and valuable nurses' work really is.

This is the complexity paradigm: diverse independent agents interact and adapt to change locally; new behavior, ideas, patterns, and structures emerge from relationships; results are often nonlinear, unpredictable, and surprising; and self-organization occurs with distributed leadership and simple rules. Once nursing leaders integrate this paradigm into their worldview, it will prompt a radical change in their approach to leadership practice, nursing care, and overall health-care delivery.

EXPANDING COMPLEXITY LEADERSHIP ROLES

There is increasing growth in the education and certification of clinical nurse leaders (CNLs) and doctors of nursing practice (DNPs). The CNL role has shown to be an especially multifaceted and valuable asset to health-care organizations. Numbers of CNLs have more than doubled since 2011, when 1,700 were reported, to approximately 5,000 as reported by the American Association of Colleges of Nursing (AACN, 2014).

Maine Medical Center (MMC) in Portland, Maine, was an early developer and champion for the CNL concept and partnered with educators from the beginning to sponsor clinical learning opportunities. Its CNLs have taken on roles of patient care, risk management, quality improvement, research, and interdisciplinary leadership, and are sought out to contribute to strategic and tactical planning. The flexibility of the role has proven valuable as a resource for meeting complex patient needs. All of these aspects of practice are enhanced by the complexity leadership perspective. The Centers for Medicare and Medicaid Services' (CMS) pay-for-performance requirements prompted MMC to track and measure actual outcomes resulting from CNL implementation and subsequent interventions. MMC reported a decrease in lengths of stay and number of readmissions, and significant improvement in specific patient outcomes required by CMS (Wilson et al, 2013).

We can see gathering evidence that approaching patient care and leadership from a complexity perspective, with knowledge of complex adaptive systems, can translate into measureable performance improvement. The evidence, such as MMC's study or the well-recognized National Institutes for Health (NIH) funded studies of nursing homes as complex adaptive systems (Anderson et al, 2003), shows that the complexity perspective can produce real performance gains. By including systems theory and complexity science in the AACN's *Essentials of Master's Education in Nursing* (2011), nursing and health care can be assured that nurses in any graduate specialty will have the knowledge to be effective complexity leaders.

LEADERSHIP STYLES AND BEHAVIOR

The history of leadership theory and practice—spanning scientific management and human relations; behavioral, trait, style, systems, situational, and transformational—has been the story of the leader's role. Early management theory put the manager in the role of being removed, outside, not part of the system but acting on the system. With each successive iteration of management theory, the role of the leader becomes less removed and more involved, not outside but within the system. Even with transformational leadership, which is relationship-based, there is still the hint of the leader inspiring others to be part of the change that the leader envisions. With complexity leadership, the journey is completed; the leader is embedded within and fully a part of the whole. When leaders are in the flow of complexity, their visions for their organizations are not theirs alone anymore.

DEVELOPMENTAL CONSIDERATIONS

The complexity leader is a transformational leader who has incorporated knowledge of complexity concepts and complex adaptive systems and who practices personal being and awareness. The journey from linear to transformational leadership is developmental, as is the further growth to complexity leadership. There is considerable evidence that there is a link between stages of adult development and stages of leadership. Transformational leaders are most frequently found in the higher stages of adult development. A later stage of ego development is Loevinger's autonomous stage. Persons at this stage can tolerate inner conflict related to competing needs, ideals, and duties. Autonomous themselves, they recognize others' need for autonomy. They value interpersonal relationships and interdependence. They embrace and cope with ambiguity (Oja, 1989).

Fisher and Torbert (1991) classify the level at which transformational leadership is possible as the *strategist*. A strategist can integrate contradiction and paradox and uses collaborative inquiry and mutual influence in leadership behavior. The next higher stage after strategist is *magician*. Magicians are more self-reflective and self-aware of feelings and actions. They view time and events from a symbolic stance, seeing patterns and the whole. The effective complexity leader may be that combination of autonomous, strategist, and magician.

Fisher and Torbert's managers were much less linear and accepted that implementation of initiatives took time and was a complex process. These managers did not try to convince others of their vision but set the stage for the process to unfold, helping people come to shared meaning. While this takes more time, these leaders believed that, in the long run, there were better outcomes and that the success in one area can roll out across the system. These managers are able to enter Stacey's zone of complexity, opening space where all the answers are not known and people are far from agreement. People with diverse mental models are encouraged to come together in relationship and to find delight in what emerges.

Weathersby (1993) offers a comprehensive description of leaders at late stages of development. These leaders are both cognitively broad and complex and can handle paradox and ambiguity. They respect individuals, practice interdependence, and understand that causation for events may be very complex and far from linear. Effective communicators, they collaborate, but they can use productive dissent for creating change. Developing others is important to them, and they are perceived by others to be transformational leaders.

Just as becoming a transformational leader is a developmental process that is seen at higher levels of ego development, there is a developmental process for the transition to complexity. The two foundations that support complexity leadership are theoretical and the personal. The theoretical foundation is knowledge and subsequent integration of complexity concepts and complex adaptive systems. The knowledge shifts one's worldview but at the same time brings the leader to the edge of leadership practice. The complexity perspective calls for a leadership style of authenticity, openness, and presence. To develop and sustain these qualities, there is the additional foundation of personal being and awareness.

PERSONAL BEING AND AWARENESS

By virtue of being embedded in the system and connected in a web of relationships, the complexity leader is more vulnerable and can feel less protected. The linear leader can afford to remain removed, self-protected, and less self-aware. For the complexity leader, personal being and awareness with self-reflective self-care practices makes the difference. With congruence and courage, even one or two nurse leaders in an organization committed to a complexity perspective can be the catalyst for positive change.

Complexity leaders are attractors, bringing new ideas and ways of leading to others, creating their own butterfly effects. Complexity leaders imagine possibilities, trust the process, discern patterns, and know that inner work affects others and their relationships. The following *Just Suppose* captures the complexity view.

JUST SUPPOSE

Just suppose...
No one can ever be an observer to any process or situation
Just suppose...
That when any one of us seeks to grow and learn or develop new insights, this elevates all of us to new levels of growth and insight
Just suppose...
That what we experience and then interpret as good or bad is neither, but just is, with meaning and purpose beyond our current comprehension
Just suppose...
That there is no one right way to do a thing or be a person
Just suppose...
We are not separate parts but our individual fields are continuous with each other, causing us all to be each other's environment
Just suppose...
That as each of us goes within to know more about ourselves, we know more about and connect better with the greater whole and each other

A CASE FOR COMPLEXITY

Rita Larson, an experienced home care administrator, assumed the position of president/CEO of Community Home and Hospice (CHH), a nonprofit agency. She knew it had a history of financial difficulties and turnovers in leadership. The mission was to provide clinically excellent home and community services to those in need, regardless of their resources. The organization had existed for more than 100 years, with rapid growth in size and complexity over the past 10 years.

Up until the late 1990s, CHH had been led by a caring, compassionate nurse who focused on relationships, both with her staff and community, rather than on costs. Due to the leader's strong community relationships, the organization was able to generate other revenues, municipal funds, donations, and bequests to make up for its operational losses The 1997 Balanced Budget Act brought sweeping changes in reimbursement to a prospective, episodic methodology, setting new rules and expectations for the industry. Within 12 months, CHH was unable to continue business as usual. Managers were not able to meet payroll or their accounts payable and began to draw on loans and lines of credit. Because the organization continued to be a value to the communities, municipal support and short-term loans allowed CHH to remain in business despite losses of $1–2 million in operations. CHH faced the same challenges as all of the home health-care industry: the threat of perpetual cuts in Medicare reimbursement and new regulations, an ever present uncertainty.

Rita's challenge was evident:

- How to reduce costs while maintaining client and staff satisfaction
- How to be effective while being efficient
- How to appear caring while cutting costs
- How to engage over 300 employees in conversation while needing to react quickly and make decisions.

The question of how to effect substantive and rapid change in a very complex adaptive system had to be addressed. Rita knew that the previous leaders had found that so much resistance from staff, the board, and the community was too great to overcome. If the prior initiatives were not sustained in the past, how would the organization learn from its past mistakes? How could she work within a complex system both internally and externally to effect permanent and positive change? How could the organization's

Continued

A CASE FOR COMPLEXITY—cont'd

board be encouraged to become part of the solution, taking a role in supporting needed changes and being proactive with staff and other stakeholders? New energy and creative initiatives were needed to keep pace with this unpredictable yet interdependent environment while maintaining a satisfied workforce and a viable organization.

Rita believed that, as the ultimate community opinion makers, the voluntary board of trustees would have to be educated about the existing external climate and new threats to its survival. Rita and her senior management team agreed that education and communication with the board must be substantive. Several outside and valued individuals, including a long-time auditor, were invited to be part of the conversations with the board. Presentations and workshops were developed, beginning with basics on the regulatory climate, the market, competition, and upcoming legislative proposals and staffing issues. Special meetings were established with trustees to avoid taking time from an already busy board agenda. Information and materials provided did not give the answers but rather elicited questions. Senior staff offered data that encouraged questions and dialogue. For example, one of the proposals for cost savings involved combining two branch offices. This allowed the board members to reflect on results of the past while contemplating what would happen if no action was taken. Several board trustees raised concerns over staff perception and use of technology. These detailed, or "how," questions were related to "what" the direction of the organization needed to become while allowing management to work with staff to determine the procedures.

Although not without concern, the board trustees and several of the senior managers who had long personal histories with the organization were able to reach a unanimous outcome to combine two offices. They left the details of where the office would be located and the layout to a committee of cross-sectional representatives from the two offices. Recognition was given to mourning the culture of the past when a dedicated nurse and office space existed in each small community. The board members could see that an array of current technology provided access to full medical records, including laboratory results, interdisciplinary team documentation, and procedures providing field staff support, so there was less need for large offices. Indeed, the staff vehicles were virtual offices.

A CASE FOR COMPLEXITY—cont'd

In her approach to this intervention, Rita used a complexity lens. She and her team helped the board understand that the organization was interdependent and had multiple stakeholders and relationships to balance. There was a shadow system that was resistant to change, whether that resistance was intentional or not, that resulted in leadership turnover and that had to be acknowledged. Good enough and simple rules kept the discussion of the board to a higher level of decision making rather than focusing on the details, which could be left to management and staff. Finally, the goal of assisting the trustees to accept the paradox that fiscal viability and client satisfaction could co-exist was met. As a complexity leader, Rita created time and space for advocacy and inquiry and diverse perspectives to be heard. With a clear focus on the mission of CHH, together they all created changes resulting in a successful conclusion to their imminent issues and challenges.

SUMMARY

Nurses are the largest group of health-care professionals. They are embedded within and throughout each and every venue of health-care delivery. Their work connects them to each and all other disciplines and to the community at large. Nurses with a complexity perspective cannot only provide excellent care at the point of service but will also be able to influence others in the system. All nurses share a responsibility to be leaders, advanced practice nurses especially so. They are the recognized leaders in their practices and organizations. Formal nurse leaders who are complexity leaders have the knowledge, power, skills, and presence to bring more and more nurses to the complexity perspective. The possibilities for effective nursing influence on health-care delivery are limitless.

Knowledge of complexity science and complex adaptive systems; a leadership style that is transformational, collaborative, self-reflective, and relationship-based; and personal being and awareness are the components of complexity leadership. The Complexity Leadership Profile is included in this chapter. This assessment helps you to discover your knowledge of complex adaptive organizations and of the actions that are unique to complexity leadership and provides an opportunity to rate your current level of personal being and awareness.

COMPLEXITY LEADERSHIP ASSESSMENT/PROFILE

The following assessment addresses the three components of the Complexity Leadership Model: knowledge of health-care organizations as complex adaptive systems, complexity leader style and action, and personal being and awareness. The goal in parts 1 and 2 is to determine your knowledge of organizations and leadership from a complexity perspective. Then, in Part 3, you will evaluate to what extent you are practicing aspects of personal being and awareness. Part 3 has no definitive answers because it is a rating scale for your personal self-reflection. After you complete all three parts, you will transfer your scores to the answer grids at the end of the assessment.

Part 1. Health-Care Organizations as Complex Adaptive Systems

Choose the answer that exemplifies the complexity science and complex adaptive systems perspective of organizations.

1. When events do not turn out as expected:
   a. there may be opportunity in this happening.
   b. the planning was not thorough enough.
   c. the person or group responsible should be identified.
   d. a review of the system is needed.
2. Where strategic planning is concerned:
   a. each step needs to be spelled out clearly.
   b. the complexity of the plan should equal the complexity of the expected results.
   c. there may not be a correlation between details and results.
   d. experts should be employed to develop the plans.
3. With regard to organization-wide planning for system change, the best philosophy to adopt is:
   a. Change the reporting structure to encourage people to change.
   b. The larger one's span of control, the harder it is to effect change.
   c. People in effective relationships can produce effective system-wide change.
   d. Informing people in detail about the change will help them accept it.
4. With regard to the most effective dissemination of information, the best philosophy to adopt is:
   a. Multiple methods and free flow of information will reach nearly everyone.
   b. Sending out information along formal reporting lines assures dissemination.

COMPLEXITY LEADERSHIP
ASSESSMENT/PROFILE—cont'd

    c. Information should be shared on a need-to-know basis to cut down on rumors.

    d. Choosing one information-sharing vehicle, e.g., a newsletter, fosters information transfer.

5. Visibility of senior management:

    a. is best accomplished by specific meetings at specific times to instill trust.

    b. is accomplished in multiple ways of relating and communicating across the organization.

    c. is best done through connections with middle management.

    d. is not expected by most people as they know how busy senior managers are.

6. The following is true about the best-run team and staff meetings:

    a. Tight control with a firm pre-published agenda gets things done.

    b. A loose and free-wheeling style gives everyone a chance to be creative and caring.

    c. There is a correlation between the duration of the meeting and the quality of the results.

    d. A well-organized agenda with time and space for new ideas to emerge is effective.

7. When two health-care organizations are in the process of merging, it is important to:

    a. decide which organization will take the lead.

    b. dissolve both organizations' plans, mission policies, and practices and start anew.

    c. create opportunities for relationship-building and sharing at all levels of the merged organization.

    d. let each organization continue as it was, with only the merged board of directors and financial/business aspects handled as one.

8. When a hospital emergency department wants to improve relationships with the community and its residents, which approach should be chosen?

    a. Hold focus-group sessions with community residents, write up the results, and disseminate to all staff.

    b. Hold focus-group sessions with community residents and, based on the feedback, write a detailed procedure for how to interact with patients.

Continued

COMPLEXITY LEADERSHIP
ASSESSMENT/PROFILE—cont'd

    c. Identify those clinicians who are not in compliance, and counsel them to reinforce the value of good community relations.

    d. Hold focus groups with community residents, and invite representatives from the community to join with staff members to develop simple, key elements of patient care and relationships.

9. A microsystem is composed of a small group of people who provide care to a subpopulation with a clinical, business, and outcome focus. The microsystem is embedded in the larger macrosytem. This is an example of which complexity concept?

    a. Diversity

    b. Attractor

    c. Fractal

    d. Butterfly effect

10. When viewing change from a complexity perspective, which of the following statements is not true?

    a. Change is not about overcoming resistance but being drawn to an attractor that exists within a pattern.

    b. Systems are the most healthy when they are in equilibrium.

    c. Small changes can have large results.

    d. Solutions cannot be transferred from one environment to another.

Part 2. Leadership Style and Action: Acting Like a Complexity Leader

Choose the action that is closest to complexity leadership behavior in each situation.

1. When contemplating a need for change in a system, structure, or process, I:

    a. gather a small group of the most knowledgeable people to draft a plan.

    b. assign a special project manager to develop the plan.

    c. confer with peers in other organizations to adopt their proven initiative.

    d. look for diverse idea and practices.

2. When forming a task force or work group, I:

    a. select from the senior leadership group.

    b. make sure the power players are in the room.

    c. select people with diverse mental models and views.

    d. look for compatibility of personality and work styles.

COMPLEXITY LEADERSHIP
ASSESSMENT/PROFILE—cont'd

3. As director of critical care and the emergency department (ED), I hear that nursing staff in the ED are complaining about recent changes in admitting procedures. My most likely approach is to:
   a. circulate at various times, observing and being open to hearing how things are going.
   b. ask their unit manager to settle them down.
   c. go to the next staff meeting and ask for feedback.
   d. ask Staff Development to re-educate them on the procedure.
4. The patient satisfaction scores for "nurses' caring and listening" have dropped for three quarters in a row. I most likely would:
   a. ignore it because the staff has recently been very stressed.
   b. disseminate the concern widely and seek ideas for improvement.
   c. ask Staff Development to hold some classes.
   d. determine which nurses are responsible.
5. I discover that the outpatient clinic staff members have fashioned their own way to process admissions and, although it seems to be easier and more comfortable for patients, it is not according to established protocol. I would most likely first:
   a. ask Staff Development to re-educate them on the proper protocol.
   b. leave them alone as it works for them.
   c. make a visit and ask them to describe their process and how it works for them.
   d. ask the unit manager to correct the situation.
6. Because of new regional health insurance regulations and a shift in the community's population, there is uncertainty about what the future holds, and there is disagreement among administration, clinical staff, and finance over whether to expand some services. As a complexity leader, my approach would be to:
   a. see what other health-care organizations have done in these circumstances.
   b. bring all the diverse parties together to share ideas.
   c. encourage senior leaders to make the decision based upon available information.
   d. do nothing until more information is known.

Continued

COMPLEXITY LEADERSHIP ASSESSMENT/PROFILE—cont'd

7. If I were to employ a collaborative approach when convening an interdisciplinary work group, I would expect:
   a. the knowledge and skills of all, beyond their discipline roles, are engaged in an interdependent, emergent process.
   b. that people would assume their usual roles and act without conscious effort and little interaction.
   c. the group to organize itself to work independently with some coordination.
   d. The group is viewed by the leaders by taking each individual and role into consideration.

8. One indication that I have developed from being a transformational to a complexity leader is:
   a. I share my values and vision so I can inspire others.
   b. with presence and patience, I set the stage for all of us to come to shared meaning.
   c. I am a role model and mentor for others across the organization.
   d. I seek others to form relationships and networks across the organization.

9. When an adverse clinical event occurs in my department that involves several disciplines, I would do all but which of the following:
   a. Encourage a collaborative after-action review.
   b. Allow for feelings and diverse opinions to be voiced and acknowledged.
   c. Turn the issue over to the risk management department.
   d. Consider what part my department or I might have played in this event.

10. As a complexity leader and change agent, I employ the complex adaptive model of organizational change. This includes all but which one of the following?
   a. A focus on significant differences, such as power, levels of expertise, cost, and quality.
   b. Setting the container, influencing the environment for self-organization and distributed control.
   c. Ensuring education is provided about benefits of the change so it will be accepted.
   d. Design transforming exchanges with many and diverse linkages and methods of communication.

COMPLEXITY LEADERSHIP ASSESSMENT/PROFILE—cont'd

Part 3. Personal Being and Awareness and Self-Reflection

Rate your self-awareness and self-care practices on a scale of 1 to 10, with 10 being most/best.

SELF-AWARENESS, SELF-CARE PRACTICE	1	2	3	4	5	6	7	8	9	10
Clarity of values										
Aware of feelings										
Less need for control, order, and certainty										
Staying centered, being present, fully listening										
Seeking and handling feedback										
Self-care, safety, nutrition, and exercise										
Centering/spiritual practice										
Family relationships										
Social relationships										
Work/life balance										

CALCULATING YOUR LEVEL OF COMPLEXITY LEADERSHIP

Part 1. Insert your answers in the table below. Give yourself 1 point for each correct answer, and count your total points. It will range from 1 to 10.

QUESTION NO.	1	2	3	4	5	6	7	8	9	10
Answers	a	c	c	a	b	d	c	d	c	b
Your Answer										

Continued

COMPLEXITY LEADERSHIP ASSESSMENT/PROFILE—cont'd

Part 1 total score_____

Part 2. Insert your answers in the table below. Give yourself 1 point for each correct answer, and count your total points. It will range from 1 to 10.

QUESTION NO.	1	2	3	4	5	6	7	8	9	10
Answers	d	c	a	b	c	b	a	b	c	c
Your Answer										

Part 2 total score _____

Part 3. Insert your rating for each self-awareness value or practice. Give yourself 0 points for ratings from 1 to 5 and 1 point for ratings from 6 to 10.

SELF-AWARENESS, SELF-CARE PRACTICE	YOUR RATING	YOUR SCORE*
Clarity of values		
Aware of feelings		
Less need for control, order, and certainty		
Staying centered, being present, fully listening		
Seeking and handling feedback		
Self-care, safety, nutrition, and exercise		
Centering/spiritual practice		
Family relationships		
Social relationships		
Work/life balance		

*0 points for 1–5 rating; 1 point for 6–10 rating.

COMPLEXITY LEADERSHIP
ASSESSMENT/PROFILE—cont'd

Part 3 total score_____

Now you can chart your Complexity Leadership profile. On the linear/complexity continuum, how close to complexity are you? Circle the total scores you calculated above, and connect to see your profile.

Complexity knowledge and perspective	1	2	3	4	5	6	7	8	9	10
Leadership style and action	1	2	3	4	5	6	7	8	9	10
Personal being and awareness	1	2	3	4	5	6	7	8	9	10

(1) Linear _____ Complexity (10)

Discovery, insight, possible action _____

QUESTIONS FOR SELF-REFLECTION

1. When I reflect on my complexity leadership profile, I find the following strengths and areas to develop.

_____

_____

_____

2. My plan for self-care practice will include the following:

_____

_____

_____

12–1 CRITICAL THINKING QUESTION

Compare and contrast the developmental stages discussed in this chapter (Oja 1989, Fisher & Torbert, 1991; Weathersby, 1993) with the leadership style and actions and personal being and awareness of the complexity leader, using complexity concepts.

REFERENCES

American Association of Colleges of Nursing (2011). *The essentials of master's education in nursing.* Retrieved March 5, 2015 from http://www.aacn.nche.edu/education-resources/MastersEssentials11.pdf

Anderson, R.A., Issel, L.M., & McDaniel, R.R. (2003). Nursing homes as complex adaptive systems: Relationships between management practice and resident outcomes. *Nurs Res 52*(1), 12-21.

Fisher, D., & Torbert, W.R. (1991). Transforming managerial practice: Beyond the achiever stage. In R.W. Woodman & W.A. Pasmore (eds.). *Research in organizational change and development,* vol. 5. Greenwich, CT: JAI Press, pp 143-173.

Oja, S.N. (1989). Teachers: Ages and stages of development. In M.L. Holly & C.S. McLoughlin (eds.), *Perspectives on teacher professional development.* London: Falmer Press, pp 119-150.

Weathersby, R. (1993). Sri Lankan manager's leadership conceptualizations as a function of ego development. In J. Demick & P.M. Miller (eds.). *Development in the workplace.* Hillsdale, NJ: Lawrence Erlbaum Associates, pp 67-89.

Wilson, L., Orff, S., Gerry, T., et al. (2013). Evolution of an innovative role: Clinical nurse leader. *Nurs Manag 21,* 175-181.

ANNOTATED BIBLIOGRAPHY

The three sections of this bibliography describe helpful resources in complexity science and organizations, leadership, and personal being and awareness.

The first section includes the texts most helpful in gaining a foundational understanding of complexity theory and its application to leadership and organizations. Section two presents contemporary leadership texts that embody complexity. The personal being and awareness literature is an array of resources for personal growth and development.

COMPLEXITY SCIENCE AND ORGANIZATIONS

Capra, F. (2002). *The hidden connections: A science for sustainable living.* New York: Anchor.
In this book, Capra pulls together the various aspects of living systems and complexity theory and applies them to current issues facing the social and economic world. The chapter on life and leadership in organizations is especially pertinent to leadership in complex adaptive systems.

Capra, F. (1997). *The web of life: A new scientific understanding of living systems.* New York: Anchor.
Capra describes scientific phenomena in an accessible manner without watering down the essential concepts. He describes the history of complexity theory, starting with systems thinking, along with various concepts of importance, including living systems and self-organization. This is an excellent primer on the science of complex systems.

Eoyang, G.H. (1997). *Coping with chaos: Seven simple tools.* Circle Pines, MN: Lagumo.
Eoyang clearly describes the elements of complexity theory and self-organization by using her approaches to leadership. She addresses butterfly effects, boundaries, transforming feedback loops, fractals, attractors, self-organization, and coupling, and she applies these to leadership

situations. This combination of complexity knowledge and practical leadership action makes this a valuable handbook.

Lewin, R., & Regine, B. (2000). *The soul at work: Using complexity science for business success.* **New York: Simon & Schuster.**
The authors describe complexity and the results of their interviews with successful businesspeople whose companies operate from a complexity perspective. They emphasize the importance of relationships and moving from command and control to a broader, more sharing, style of leadership. Reading about these companies and how they use complexity brings the theory to life and offers valuable insights into how to practice complexity leadership.

Lindberg, C., Nash, S., & Lindberg, C. (eds.). (2008). *On the edge: Nursing in the age of complexity.* **Scotts Valley, CA: CreateSpace.**
Nursing is in the forefront of applying complexity principles to health-care leadership. This book is a compilation of contributed chapters that describe complexity and its application to health care and that also offer several examples of models and practices in use today by nurse leaders. Topics include nursing theory, research, leadership, and family interventions. Theirs is an excellent complexity science primer as well.

Stacey, R. (1996). *Complexity and creativity in organizations.* **San Francisco: Berrett-Koehler Publishers.**
This groundbreaking work introduced complexity thinking to organizations. It includes important material related to organizations as complex adaptive systems. Stacey presents models for understanding adaptive feedback networks, learning systems, and self-organization as well as implications for applying complexity theory to organizations. The book also includes an excellent glossary of terms.

Stacey, R. (2007). *Strategic management and organisational dynamics: The challenge of complexity* **(5th ed.). New York: Prentice Hall.**
This book is a comprehensive treatment of the various philosophies and theories about organizational systems and, more importantly, how management and leaders think about their organizations. Stacey traces the history and progression of organizational management approaches and how they change over time. Along with an excellent review of previous paradigms, Stacey elucidates how complexity concepts such as limit of control, unpredictability, and critical systems thinking contribute to effective organizational leadership.

Wheatley, M.J. (2006). *Leadership and the new science: Discovering order in a chaotic world* **(3rd ed.). San Francisco: Berrett-Koehler Publishers.**
This seminal work had enormous impact on business and organizational leadership. Wheatley was one of the first authors to connect the new concepts found in science to the organizational management

world. Her writing style and enthusiasm for her topic brought science to management in believable and poetic fashion, causing readers to think of control and order from a new perspective.

Zimmerman, B., Lindberg, C., & Plesek, P. (2001). *Edgeware: Insights from complexity science for health care leaders* (2nd ed.). VHA, Inc.

This was the first book to apply complexity theory to health-care leadership. The authors were experienced health-care leaders who first transmitted these ideas to their colleagues. The book describes and explains complexity and then presents many activities and examples using real-life situations. The authors provide tools for health-care leaders to help their teams start thinking like complexity leaders and navigating today's many challenges.

LEADERSHIP

Brofman, O. & Beckstrom, R.A. (2006). *The starfish and the spider: The unstoppable power of leaderless organizations.* New York: Penguin Group.

The authors provide a contemporary view of organizations that are decentralized and successful. They discuss several examples of leaderless organizations, such as Alcoholics Anonymous and the Internet. These are samples of self-organized systems, local level activity, and open systems, all open to change. The book includes real-world examples of complexity in action.

Goleman, D., Boyatzis, R., & McKee, A. (2002). *Primal leadership: Learning to lead with emotional intelligence.* Boston: Harvard Business Publishing.

Building on earlier works on emotional intelligence, the authors discuss leadership. Primal leadership is emotionally compelling. Resonant leaders with emotional intelligence connect with others in rich relationships, the power of their actions swaying others. The authors have a repertoire that consists of visioning, coaching, affiliation, being democratic, pace setting, and commanding when needed. Resonant and dissonant leadership styles are discussed. The book offers a process to become a successful primal leader with emotional intelligence.

Heifetz, R., Grashow, A., Linsky, M. (2009). *The practice of adaptive leadership: Tools and tactics for changing your organization and the world.* Cambridge, MA: Harvard Business Press.

Adaptive leadership represents a form of leadership based on complexity. The authors distinguish between adaptive leadership and technical leadership, which includes the transactional, more linear aspects of leading. Both are needed, and knowing which is required is essential. Adaptive leadership entails mobilizing people to tackle challenges and to thrive. The components of diversity and experimentation are inherent in bringing about change and meeting challenges. This is a valuable adjunct to complexity thinking and leadership.

Lipmanowicz, H., & McCandless, K. (2013). *The surprising power of liberating structures: Simple rules to unleash a culture of innovation.* Seattle, WA: Liberating Structures Press.

Lipmanowicz and McCandless provide a rich and much needed resource to leaders and teachers of leadership who want to use the concepts of nonlinearity in leaderships, not only in theory but in practice. This makes for a congruency between what is presented and used, and what is taught theoretically. The text is replete with theory, but of a more practical nature, there are well-described exercises and many examples, some of which are real-life situations provided by guest authors. This text is the most practical and essential adjunct to leading and teaching in the complexity paradigm.

Mindell, A. (1992). *The leader as martial artist: An introduction to deep democracy.* San Francisco: Harper.

Based on field theory and process-oriented psychology, and informed by Jungian and Eastern concepts, this book gives new insights into leading in conflict-laden situations. Mindell suggests field interventions when working with groups and being in the role of facilitator. He explores such leadership meta-skills as compassion, working with group energy, and developing a sense of detachment. Mindell proposes deeper-level skills for the centered complexity leader.

Neal, J. (2013). *Creating enlightened organizations: Four gateways to spirit at work.* New York: Palgrave Macmillan.

Judi Neal, author of *Edgewalkers,* continues her work with spirit in the workplace with this presentation of four gateways to spirit at work. These are: creating personal transformation, developing enlightened leaders and team, creating organizational transformation and joining the global consciousness shift. Neal's spirit at work is not about specific religions but the belief in and connection to a transcendent reality. Her approach offers valuable reflections and suggestions for any leader, team, or organization to work with enhanced spirit and effectiveness.

Schein, E. (2013). *Humble inquiry: The gentle art of asking instead of telling.* San Francisco: Berrett-Koehler Publishers.

Edgar Schein's long and respected career in teaching and consulting in management, especially concerning culture and leadership, prompted this text. He came to believe that building positive relationships is essential to building better organizations. He discusses methods of humble inquiry that require much less telling and more asking. He describes our Western culture of task orientation combined with rank and power as holding us back from getting the ideas and information needed to improve our organizations. With excellent examples and self-reflection questions, this text truly enriches organizational leadership and communication literature.

Shelton, C. (1999). *Quantum leaps: Seven skills for workplace re-creation.* St. Louis: Elsevier/Butterworth-Heinemann.
In her leadership model, Shelton applies the concepts of quantum science and complexity. Hers was an early publication to directly relate new science in a concrete way to contemporary organizations. The quantum skills are seeing intentionally, thinking paradoxically, feeling vitally alive, knowing intuitively, acting responsibly, trusting life, and being in relationship. The book investigates aspects of organizational leadership and personal growth.

PERSONAL BEING AND AWARENESS

Birx, E. (2002). *Healing Zen: Awakening to a life of wholeness and compassion while caring for yourself and others.* New York: Viking.
Ellen Birx is a registered nurse with a Zen practice. She uses her experience as a nurse to illustrate examples of healing and self-care. Dr. Birx discusses presence, breathing, energy, confidence, acceptance, appreciation, and balance. Nurse leaders can find valuable help for personal growth and nursing practice.

Conner, J. (2008). *Writing down your soul: How to activate and listen to the extraordinary voice within.* Newburyport, MA: Conari Press.
Janet Conner offers a unique way to maintain a journal. She asserts that by setting intention and following a process, you can activate and listen to the voice within. In other words, your inner-voice wisdom can be tapped with journaling. Connor lays out this process in four steps: show up, open up, listen up, and follow up. This book can be an effective tool for getting in touch with how you really feel and can serve as a form of meditative practice.

Crum, T. (2006). *Three deep breaths: Finding power and purpose in a stressed-out world.* San Francisco: Berrett-Koehler.
The author of *The Magic of Conflict,* Crum offers insight into finding power and purpose in a stressed-out world through telling the story of Angus. Angus learns about the centering breath, the possibility breath, and the discovery breath. Centering practices that focus on breathing can bring balance, purpose, and power to one's life.

Jacobs, J. (2007). *In a pickle? Nourishing recipes & food for thought.* Peterborough, NH: Infinite Strategies.
This book is at once light-hearted and deeply wise. It has great ideas for cooking your way out of everyday "pickles." Jacobs provides recipes, such as lemonade, and then wisdom to change your attitude to make lemons into lemonade. Chicken noodle soup is used as a metaphor for groups. Several difficult topics are covered in this book of recipes and insight.

Ringer, J. (2006). *Unlikely teachers: Finding the hidden gifts in daily conflict.*
   Portsmouth, NH: OnePoint Press
Judy Ringer teaches conflict management and has a Black Belt in Aikido martial arts. In this series of stories, she uses Aikido to explain how to become more conscious of how people invent their lives from moment to moment, by transforming challenges into opportunities. Each story illustrates the learning derived from a difficult or conflict situation. Ringer illustrates progression from resistance to a conflict, to connecting with it, and to action, discovering new power and finally recognizing the conflict as a teacher.

Ruiz, D.M. (1997). *The four agreements: A practical guide to personal freedom.*
   San Rafael, CA: Amber-Allen Publishing.
This book has become a widely used vehicle for personal growth and dealing with self and others. Study groups have been built around the four agreements, which are: (1) be impeccable in your word, (2) do not take anything personally, (3) do not make assumptions, and (4) always do your best. These have very relevant applicability to effective personal and professional leadership.

Ruiz, D.M., Ruiz, D.J., & Mills, J. (2010). *The fifth agreement: A practical guide to
   self-mastery.* San Raphael, CA: Amber-Allen Publishing.
As the title suggests, this book is a continuation of *The Four Agreements*. The fifth agreement addresses self-acceptance and acceptance of others. It gives considerable attention to the concept that each individual sees the world from that individual's perspective, different from all others. This is similar to Stacey's diversity of mental models. With this understanding, the leader is more likely to embrace various viewpoints and look for ways to bring everyone together for the greater idea rather than try to convert others to the leader's point of view. Once you accept the fifth agreement, you can express your own views with more comfort.

INDEX

Note: Page numbers followed by "b," "f," and "t" indicate boxes, figures, and tables, respectively.